SECOND AND THIRD
GENERATION
ANTIPSYCHOTICS

A COMPREHENSIVE HANDBOOK

RYAN S. O'DELL
THOMAS L. SCHWARTZ

authorHOUSE®

AuthorHouse™
1663 Liberty Drive
Bloomington, IN 47403
www.authorhouse.com
Phone: 1 (800) 839-8640

Published by AuthorHouse   08/09/2016

ISBN: 978-1-5246-1971-8 (sc)
ISBN: 978-1-5246-1972-5 (hc)
ISBN: 978-1-5246-1973-2 (e)

Library of Congress Control Number: 2016911953

Print information available on the last page.

O'Dell, R.S.[1] and Schwartz, T.L.[2]

[1]MD/PhD Program, SUNY Upstate Medical University, Syracuse, NY, 13210, USA

[2]The Department of Psychiatry, SUNY Upstate Medical University, 328 Psychiatry and Behavioral Sciences Building, 713 Harrison Street, Syracuse, NY 13210, USA

Author Contribution Statement

RSO and TLS conducted a comprehensive review of literature, wrote, and edited the manuscript.

Competing Interests Statement

The authors declare no competing financial interests.

TABLE OF CONTENTS

LIST OF TABLES

LIST OF ABBREVIATIONS

FGA   First generation antipsychotic
EPS   Extrapyradmial symptoms
SGA   Second generation antipsychotics
FDA   Food and drug administration
MDD   Major depressive disorder
TD   Tardive dyskinesia
SRI   Serotonin reuptake inhibitor
NRI   Norepinephrine reuptake inhibitor
HAM-D   Hamilton Rating Scale for Depression
BDNF   Brain-derived neurotrophic factor
GAD   Generalized anxiety disorder
HAM-A   Hamilton Rating Scale for Anxiety
PD   Panic disorder
SAD   Social anxiety disorder
PTSD   Post-traumatic stress disorder
NMS   Neuroleptic malignant syndrome
CYP   Cytochrome P450
ER   Extended release
RCT   Randomized controlled trial
NET   Norepinephrine transporter
SERT   Serotonin transporter
MADRS   Montgomery-Asberg Depression Rating Scale
CGI-S   Clinical Global Impression-Severity of Illness
YMRS   Young Mania Rating Scale
SDS   Sheehan Disability Scale
XR   Slow release
TGA   Third generation antipsychotic
bid   Twice daily
AUC   Area under the curve
D2   Dopamine D2 receptor

D3	Dopamine D3 receptor
5-HT1a	Serotonin 1a receptor
5-HT2a	Serotonin 2a receptor
5-HT2c	Serotonin 2c receptor
5-HT6	Serotonin 6 receptor
5-HT7	Serotonin 7 receptor
α1	Alpha adrenergic 1 receptor
α2	Alpha adrenergic 2 receptor
M1	Muscarinic acetylcholine 1 receptor
H1	Histamine 1 receptor

FOREWORD

The second and third generation antipsychotics (SGA/TGA)
have a wide range of approved treatment indications, including
schizophrenia, bipolar mania and depression, major depressive
disorder, and autism. Each medication in this class varies not only
in their approved treatment indications, but demonstrate a diverse
spectrum of off-label uses, applicability to special populations
(adults vs. adolescents), and treatment regiment (monotherapy
vs. adjunct therapy). This is largely a consequence of the unique
pharmacodynamic profile of each agent, which often necessitates
the employment of unique dosing strategies across the treatment of
these varied psychiatric disorders.

With the advent of three new SGAs in recent years (lurasidone
2011, brexpiprazole 2015, and cariprazine 2015), two of which
are partial dopamine receptor agonists (now coined TGA by
the authors), we aim to review data relevant to the treatment
indications, off-label use, and dosing strategies of all current agents
using an evidence-based approach. Where definitive data are
lacking, theoretical commentary based upon pharmacodynamic
profiles and less stringent clinical trials will be employed. These
agents are characterized by a diverse range of clinical applications,
both FDA approved and off-label. This definitive text is current and
up to date regarding all available agents and should provide mental
health prescribers with the tools necessary to optimize treatment
based upon patient diagnosis, proper antipsychotic selection, and
implementation of an appropriate dosing strategy (low, middle,
or high ranges), thereby striking an essential balance between
treatment efficacy and patient tolerability.

Ryan Stephen O'Dell

Thomas L. Schwartz

INTRODUCTION

The typical antipsychotics, also known as first generation antipsychotics (FGA), were developed in the 1950s and were solely approved to treat acute psychosis and manage chronic psychotic disorders, primarily schizophrenia. All FGAs are known to exert their pharmacologic effects via postsynaptic antagonism of the dopamine D2 receptor, with a requirement of at least 65.0% receptor occupancy for antipsychotic efficacy[1]. As D2 receptor occupancy increases, antipsychotic efficacy tends to increase, but so does the risk for side effects, including hyperprolactinemia (70%) and extrapyramidal symtpoms (EPS; dystonia, akathisia, parkinsonism, neuroleptic malignant syndrome, and tardive dyskinesia at 80%). High potency FGAs (fluphenazine, thiothixene, and haldoperidol), dosed in 1.0 to 10.0s of milligrams, have a much greater risk for these side effects due to their relatively high affinity for D2 receptors as their main pharamacodynamic profile. Low potency FGAs however (chlorpromazine and thioridazine), dosed in 100.0s of milligrams, have lower EPS risk profiles (due to their higher affinities for histaminic and muscarinic receptors) and demonstrate a greater risk of sedation, orthostatic hypotension, and weight gain. As dosage increases, so does antipsychotic efficacy, again through D2 receptor blockade and subsequent attenuation of dopaminergic hyperactivity in the mesolimbic DA pathway[2,3]. In the past, the clinical goal was to increase FGA dosages until psychotic symptoms abated, oftentimes within rapid timeframes (neuroleptization). With the advent of the second generation antipsychotics (SGA) in the mid-1990s however, came a more complex pharmacodynamic profile, thereby necessitating a more intricate dosing strategy for some agents. This manuscript will review and discuss the clinical dosing strategies based upon clinical data, the pharmacodynamic, and pharmacokinetic profiles of the eleven currently FDA approved SGAs.

Due to the unique pharmacodynamic nature of each SGA, dosing and cross-titration strategies have become significantly more complex. Unlike FGAs, with which physicians could use an equivalency table of relative affinity values for immediate 24-hour cross-titration[4,5], SGAs often require a more gradual cross-titration approach, as setting up equivalencies is fraught with complications as more than sole D2 affinity must be accounted for. There are also often discrepancies between FDA recommended dosing approaches and clinical practice. This is primarily a consequence of risperidone's initial approval in the early 1990s for the treatment of schizophrenia and the recommended rapid escalation dosing strategy of reaching 6.0 mg in 3 days. Despite FDA assurance and data supporting low EPS rates, clinicians quickly noticed much higher rates of EPS with this dosing strategy, leading to problems with patient compliance. Although a slower titration strategy attenuates side effect risks, clinicians became cautious, often under-dosing and possibly curbing antipsychotic effectiveness[6]. This conservative approach unfortunately carried over into the subsequently approved SGAs, including olanzapine, quetiapine, ziprasidone, and aripiprazole. With the accumulation of a larger evidence base and clinical experience however, physicians have become more comfortable with the full use of the SGA dosing range[7]. In fact, some psychiatric centers often use doses much higher than those recommended in the initial approval[6,8-12]. Ideally, the full ranges of the three newest SGAs (lurasidone, brexpiprazole, and cariprazine) will be utilized.

Dosing of SGAs became more complex with the investigation and subsequent FDA approval for treatment of bipolar mania, bipolar depression, and unipolar major depressive disorder (MDD). In regard to bipolar mania, FDA recommendations were akin to 'loading' strategies, dosing SGAs very high within rapid timeframes to achieve antimanic efficacy. It therefore seemed that bipolar dosing was higher than that for schizophrenia, which was counterintuitive to most clinicians. For antidepressant properties (either as adjunctive or monotherapy), recommended initiation and target doses are much lower as compared to antipsychotic and antimanic doses. Each SGA has not only a unique pharmacodynamic profile, but also unique dosing strategies based on poly-receptor affinities and the disorder being treated.

Similar to FGAs, the SGAs act as antagonists of the D2 receptor[3], ultimately exerting their antipsychotic efficacy similarly through the attenuation of dopaminergic hyperactivity in the mesolimbic pathway. As a general rule, SGAs with higher binding affinities could be assigned an initial higher potency allowing them to achieve their antipsychotic effects at lower dosages and likely cause EPS to a greater degree. The SGAs loosely ranked from highest to lowest D2 affinity (assessed by Ki) are as follows: aripiprazole, lurasidone, brexpiprazole, and cariprazine (< 1.0 nM); risperidone, paliperidone, ziprasidone, iloperidone, and asenapine (1.0 nm to 10.0 nm); olanzapine (10.0 nM to 100.0 nM); and quetiapine (>100.0 nM)[13-22]. Unfortunately, as each binding affinity study differs in regard to source (cloned vs. brain, i.e. *in vitro* vs. *in vivo*), species (human vs. rat), and ligand used, this list can only represent a rough approximation of D2 binding affinities of the SGAs. Furthermore, aripiprazole, brexpiprazole, and cariprazine may have high affinity, but are partial agonists. They have a greater affinity to bind D2, but do not fully block D2 activity as such[23].

In addition to D2 receptor antagonism, most SGAs also demonstrate high binding affinities and antagonistic effects at serotonin-2a (5-HT2a) receptors[3,24]. 5-HT2a receptor blockade results in increased dopamine and norepinephrine release into the synaptic cleft. Although this mechanism of action may seem counterproductive to therapeutic effects on psychosis, increased neurotransmission in the mesocortical, nigrostriatal, and tuberoinfundibular pathways may alleviate iatrogenic, bradykinetic negative symptoms, and simultaneously attenuate

EPS by preferentially allowing DA activity to continue in the nigrostriatal pathway. In the mesocortical pathway, dopaminergic *hypo*activity is believed to be the root cause of both the negative and cognitive symptoms in schizophrenia[3,25-27], and therefore increased dopaminergic transmission via 5-HT2a antagonism may aide in the treatment of these symptoms. D2 receptor blockade in the nigrostriatal pathway is known to be responsible for the EPS common to antipsychotic medications[3,28-30], and 5-HT2a antagonism thereby decreases the risk of such side effects by increasing dopamine/norepinephrine release here. Similarly, D2 antagonism in the tuberoinfundibular pathway results in hyperprolactinemia[3,31], and these side effects are often attenuated via simultaneous 5-HT2a antagonism in this pathway. Interestingly, as there are fewer 5-HT2a receptors in the mesolimbic pathway, the antipsychotic properties of the SGAs (via D2 antagonism) are preserved[3]. Taken together, this dual receptor antagonism allows for the selective attenuation of dopaminergic hyperactivity in the mesolimbic system necessary for the treatment of the positive/psychotic symptoms of schizophrenia, while lowering the overall risk for EPS. It is this decreased risk of tardive dyskinesia (TD) and EPS for which the 'atypical' antipsychotics were named[3,32].

Another hypothesis for the atypical properties of these drugs suggests that dopamine blockade lasts just long enough to exert antipsychotic efficacy, but not so long as to result in EPS. This is known as the 'hit-and-run' or 'rapid dissociation' hypothesis[1,3,33-35]. According to this theory, the 'atypicality' of SGAs is due to 'loose' D2 binding and rapid dissociation, as opposed to the mechanistic 5-HT2a antagonism in the nigrostriatal pathway. Binding ('hit' phase) and subsequent blockade of the D2 receptor is responsible for the antipsychotic effects in the mesolimbic system, while a prolonged 'hit' phase in the nigrostriatal pathway results in EPS. After ligand dissociation ('run' phase), natural dopamine can flood the synaptic cleft before the next dose, and this is believed to prevent the development of motor side effects. Although it is believed that some SGAs demonstrate looser binding, rapid dissociation from the D2 receptor, and shorter half lives (as compared to FGAs), there are definitive differences within the SGA class[35]. For example, as rapid dissociation occurs more readily with lower-potency, shorter half-life medications, drugs such as clozapine and quetiapine (dosed at higher milligrams and lower D2 binding affinities) are characterized by lower rates of motor side effects. Higher relative potency agents (such as aripiprazole, lurasidone, brexpiprazole, and cariprazine) bind the D2 receptor more tightly, and are generally correlated with higher rates of EPS. Olanzapine, a drug of intermediate D2 potency, falls somewhere in the middle. Therefore, SGAs (especially those of high D2 binding affinity) require careful dosing to maximize antipsychotic efficacy while minimizing EPS and motor side effects.

Despite a decreased risk for EPS, the SGAs carry a greater risk for weight gain, diabetes mellitus, hypercholesterolemia, and hypertension as compared to FGAs[36-38]. This is known as the metabolic syndrome. Although SGAs have demonstrated altered metabolic control and increased appetite[39], the exact pharmacologic mechanisms responsible for these side effects remain unknown, and certain SGAs are more prone to these side effects than others. In addition to the dual D2/5-HT2a antagonism common to all SGAs, each drug in this class has a unique receptor binding profile that theoretically may convey increased metabolic risk. It is well known that antagonism of the hypothalamic histamine H1 receptor can lead to increased hunger and caloric intake, eventually resulting in weight gain and potential development of the metabolic syndrome[3,40-45]. In addition, antagonism of the 5-HT2c receptor has been shown to increase feeding activity and adiposity[46-49]. It is therefore postulated that SGAs with greater affinity for these two receptors may lead to increased weight gain and greater risk of the metabolic syndrome. Finally, the SGAs all differ with respect to their SRI, NRI, 5-HT1A, 5-HT2a/c, 5-HT3, 5-HT6, and 5-HT7 activities and affinities, all of which may convey important antidepressant properties as well. The next section will specifically discuss the nuances of each SGA using an evidence-based approach, reviewing their individual treatment indications, off-label uses, dosing strategies, and side-effect profiles from a pharmacodynamic perspective.

CHAPTER 1

THE '-DONES'

RISPERIDONE

The first modern atypical antipsychotic, risperidone, was approved for the treatment of schizophrenia in 1993. It is currently approved for both the acute and maintenance treatment of schizophrenia (in adults and adolescents aged 13-17 years), the acute phase of bipolar I disorder (mania or mixed episode) either as monotherapy or adjunct treatment with lithium or valproate, and irritability associated with autistic disorder[50] (**Table 1**). This drug is absorbed consistently after ingestion, with an oral bioavailability of 70.0% and a peak plasma concentration within 1-2 hours[50] (**Table 4**). With respect to dosing strategies in adults with schizophrenia, a typical initial dose is 1.0-2.0 mg/day, with a target dose of 4.0-6.0 mg/day and a maximum dose of 16.0 mg/day[3,50,51] (**Table 1**). Adolescents should be started at 0.5 mg/day and titrated to a daily dose of 3.0 mg/day. Dosing adjustments should not occur at intervals less than 24 hours and at increments of 1.0-2.0 mg for adults and 0.5-1.0 mg for adolescents. There are no current guidelines for to the long-term use of risperidone (beyond 8 weeks) in adolescents with schizophrenia. However, a recent open-label, multicenter study demonstrated risperidone maintenance treatment was efficacious and well tolerated over 6 to 12 months in adolescents with schizophrenia.[52]

In adults with bipolar mania, initiation doses are typically higher and utilize a loading strategy (2.0-3.0 mg/day with a maximum dose of 6.0 mg/day; **Table 1**)[50,53]. In pediatric populations, a starting dose of 0.5 mg/day with a target of 2.5 mg/day and maximum dose of 6.0 mg/day is recommended. As these recommendations were based on short-term, 3-week trials of antimanic efficacy, there are no current guidelines or approvals for the use of risperidone as maintenance therapy for bipolar mania.

Lastly, in regard to the treatment of irritability and aggression associated with autism (5-18 years of age), lower initiation doses of 0.25 mg/day (patients < 20.0 kg) and 0.5 mg/day (patients > 20.0 kg) are recommended[50,54] (**Table 1**). The titration strategy is slow, with a minimum of four days at the starting dose, with increases in increments of 0.25-0.5 mg at 14-day intervals. Average efficacious doses range between 0.5 mg/day and 2.5 mg/day, with a maximum daily dose of 3 mg/day.

For all treatment indications, the dosing of risperidone (or any atypical antipsychotic) should be individualized and should demonstrate a careful balance between symptom alleviation and patient tolerability. Once clinical efficacy has been maintained, physicians must always consider a gradual taper or further titration of the dosage to optimize this balance between symptom efficacy and safety. Based upon clinical trials and clinical experience, it therefore appears that higher doses of risperidone are required for the treatment of psychotic or manic symptoms, while lower doses can be used to curb irritation in children with autism. This antipsychotic attenuation is most likely due to higher (> 65.0%) D2 receptor occupancy and antagonism in the mesolimbic pathway at higher doses, while at lower doses, there is little receptor occupancy and therefore less antipsychotic effect[1,3]. This is a property common to all SGAs.

Although not approved for the treatment of depression or anxiety, there exists a fair amount of evidence supporting the efficacy of risperidone in these psychiatric illnesses. The doses are often lower, suggesting that D2 receptor antagonism is not the responsible mechanism. The efficacy of risperidone in the treatment of MDD was first described in case reports[55-57], and there are currently five randomized, placebo-controlled trials suggesting low-dose risperidone as successful augmentation therapy in treatment resistant depression. The oldest of these studies in 2006 demonstrated that low-dose risperidone augmentation (0.25-2.0 mg/day) to citalopram (40.0-60.0 mg/day) in patients with treatment resistant depression improved both the relapse rate (56.1% vs.

64.1%) and median time to relapse (97 days vs. 56 days)[58]. In this study, patients were treated with 4-6 weeks of citalopram monotherapy, followed by 4-6 weeks of open-label risperidone augmentation, and finally a 24-week double-blind continuation phase. A smaller but similarly designed trial also found a trending, but non-significant decrease in the relapse rate (56.0% vs. 65.0%) with low-dose risperidone augmentation[59]. In 2007, a six-week trial of risperidone augmentation (1.0-2.0 mg/day) demonstrated a statistically significant reduction in depressive symptoms, an increase in both response rate and remission, and improvements in Hamilton rating scale for depression (HAM-D) scores[60]. A randomized crossover study in 2008 also suggested that low-dose risperidone (0.5-2.0 mg/day) was especially efficacious in the treatment of suicidality[61]. Finally, the most recent of these five studies (2009) provided further evidence for the use of low-dose risperidone (0.5-3.0 mg/day) as a therapeutic option for treatment resistant depression, demonstrating both faster responses and improved quality of life in a short-term, 4-week augmentation trial[62]. Mechanistically, 5-HT2a antagonism (similar to that seen with the antidepressants nefazodone and trazodone) may explain this antidepressant efficacy.

Other, less well-controlled investigations have also demonstrated such antidepressive efficacy of low-dose risperidone. For example, a recent study demonstrated significant improvements in both depressive and psychotic symptoms when risperidone (2.0 mg/day) was used as an adjunct (to citalopram or venlafaxine XR) for the short-term treatment of MDD with psychotic features[63]. In addition, there was similar efficacy with either quetiapine (300.0 mg/day) or olanzapine (15.0 mg/day) adjunctive therapy. However, larger controlled trials are needed to compare the long-term efficacy and tolerability of risperidone in the treatment of MDD, both with and without psychotic features. Finally, a small, open-label study suggested risperidone augmentation to sertraline improved symptoms in patients with sertraline-resistant depression and promoted increased levels of brain derived neurotrophic factor (BDNF)[64]. It is plausible that increased levels of BDNF, a known mediator of neuronal growth, differentiation, and synaptogenesis[65], alleviates depressive symptoms through improved neuronal connections and/or neurotransmission[66]. Abnormalities in BDNF signaling have also been linked to the etiologies of both schizophrenia[67-69] and mood disorders[67,70,71], further suggesting that the use of pharmacologic agents which modify BDNF signaling (i.e. low-dose risperidone) may prove helpful in these disorders.

In regard to the treatment of anxiety disorders, early investigations suggested low-dose adjunctive risperidone (0.5-1.5 mg/day) might be a useful tool in the management of generalized anxiety disorder (GAD) patients[72]. Although this double-blind, placebo-controlled study demonstrated significant improvements in Hamilton Rating Scale for Anxiety (HAM-A) scores after 5 weeks of adjunctive treatment, the higher response rates in the treatment group failed to achieve statistical significance. In addition, a brief (8 week) open-label study suggested augmentation with low-dose risperidone (0.25-3.0 mg/day) might be a useful option for the treatment of panic disorder (PD), GAD, or social anxiety disorder (SAD), as assessed by a significant reduction in anxiety symptoms[73]. This study however had no control or placebo group. A double-blind, prospective, placebo-controlled, randomized 4 week study however demonstrated similarly improved outcomes in the treatment of GAD with either adjunctive risperidone or placebo[74]. In addition, a more recent placebo-controlled trial found 8 weeks of risperidone monotherapy (0.5-4.0 mg/day) was not effective for the treatment of bipolar patients with comorbid PD or GAD[75]. Overall, the currently available data suggests that risperidone may have greater antidepressant than anxiolytic properties.

These studies shed light on a common theme in this review: the complex pharmacodynamics of risperidone (and by extension all SGAs) allows these agents to function at differing doses to treat varied symptoms and syndromes. In this case, risperidone can be used at higher doses to treat psychotic and/or manic symptoms, primarily through its D2 antagonism in the mesolimbic pathway[2,3]. At lower doses (< 3.0 mg/day), it appears useful for the treatment of depressive symptoms (and to a lesser extent, anxiety), albeit as augmentation strategies. Although risperidone demonstrates a high binding affinity for the D2 receptor (**Table 5**), at lower doses, there is presumably lower D2 blockade. It is therefore believed that this antidepressant efficacy is mediated via antagonism of the 5-HT2a receptor, for which risperidone has an even higher affinity (**Table 5**). As previously discussed, 5-HT2a receptor antagonism and the subsequent increased release of dopamine and norepinephrine in the nigrostriatal pathway decreases the risk for EPS[3]. In the mesocortical pathway, this increase in dopamine is suggested to not only alleviate the negative symptoms of schizophrenia, but also promote improved concentration, attention, and executive functioning[3,25-27]. These 'cognitive' symptoms are also common in depressive and anxiety disorders and therefore this selective promotion of dopaminergic activity may be responsible for the aforementioned antidepressant effects. In addition, it is believed that antagonism at the α2-adrenergic receptor (for which risperidone has a high affinity; **Table 5**) contributes to antidepressant efficacy of this drug via enhancement of terminal norepinephrine release[76,77]. Risperidone also has some affinity for the 5-HT7 receptor (**Table 5**), and antagonism at this site has been shown to mediate antidepressant-like effect in animal models of MDD and in humans may improve cognition and circadian function[78,79].

Based upon the pharamacodynamic profile of risperidone, it should also be noted that patients should be monitored for dizziness, sedation, and hypotension, due to the high affinity and antagonism for α1-adrenergic receptors (**Table 5**). This α1 antagonism may also theoretically reduce nightmares, similar to the use of prazosin for the treatment of nightmares in patients with post-traumatic stress disorder (PTSD). Risperidone's moderate affinity for, and antagonism to, the histamine H1 receptor (**Table 5**) should also prompt clinicians to monitor for sedation and increased cardiometabolic side effects. Despite a high affinity for 5-HT2a receptors in the tuberoinfundibular pathway, risperidone has a higher risk of hyperprolactinemia than other SGAs[80]. It has been proposed that poor penetration of the blood-brain barrier of both risperidone and its metabolite (9-hydroxy-risperidone) might contribute to this drug's high propensity to cause hyperprolactinemia (and the subsequent amenorrhea, galactorrhea, and sexual side effects)[81-83]. Lastly, physicians should also be aware of the potential SGA class-effect risks including: metabolic syndrome (diabetes, hyperglycemia, dyslipidemia, and weight gain), leukopenia, neutropenia, agranulocytosis, neuroleptic malignant syndrome (NMS), suicidal behavior, cerebrovascular adverse reactions (in elderly populations with dementia), priapism, body temperature dysregulation, venous thromboembolism, rebound psychosis upon withdrawal, seizure induction, increased sensitivity in patients with Parkinson's disease/dementia with Lewy bodies, and prolongation of the QT interval[50]. These class-effect risks are given for all SGAs, but the specific risks for each SGA may very immensely. For example, the newer SGAs tend to have less metabolic risks but carry the same class warning.

Lastly, as risperidone is a known substrate of cytochrome P450 (CYP)2D6 (**Table 4**), concomitant use of enzyme inducers (carbamazepine, phenytoin, rifampin, and phenobarbital) should necessitate an approximate doubling of the patient's usual dose[50]. Co-administration of CYP2D6 inhibitors (fluoxetine, paroxetine, and quinidine) should be accompanied by a reduction of risperidone to approximately half of the usual dose (not to exceed 8.0 mg/day).

PALIPERIDONE

Paliperidone, the active metabolite or risperidone, appeared on the market in the US in 2006, and is currently approved for the treatment of psychosis related to schizophrenia (in both adults and adolescents) and as either monotherapy or adjunct treatment to mood stabilizers for schizoaffective disorder in adults[84] (**Table 1**). It has an oral bioavailability of 28.0% (42.0% with food) and a peak plasma concentration of 24 hours[84] (**Table 4**). Regarding dosing strategies, an average initial dose in adults with schizophrenia or schizoaffective disorder is 6.0 mg/day (no initial dose titration is needed) with a maximum dose of 12.0 mg/day (**Table 1**). If dose titration is required, increments of 3.0 mg/day at intervals of greater than 5 days is recommended[84]. Similar to risperidone, lower doses are recommended in the treatment of adolescents (12-17 years) with schizophrenia, with a 3.0 mg/day starting dose and a maximum of 6.0 mg/day[84].

In regard to the off-label use of paliperidone augmentation in treatment resistant depression, only a single case report is currently available[85]. This case report describes a 54-year old female who received 3.0 mg/day of paliperidone in addition to venlafaxine-XR 37.5 mg/day (previously treated with venlafaxine 225.0 mg/day 3 weeks prior to augmentation). Within six days, there was reported improvement of depressive symptoms (mood, sleep, energy level) and a 40.0% decreased in her HAM-D score, and within 2 weeks, the patient achieved full remission (maintained for 4 months). A MEDLINE search suggests no findings for the use of paliperidone in the treatment of anxiety disorders.

As an active metabolite of risperidone, paliperidone displays a similar pharmacodynamic profile to that of its parent product (**Table 5**), and also shares its mechanism for its antipsychotic properties at therapeutic doses. Although there is an extremely limited evidence base (one case report), the similar binding affinities to and antagonism for D2/5-HT2a receptors suggests paliperidone might have an ability to treat depressive symptoms when used as a low-dose, augmentation strategy. In addition, its affinity for the histamine H1 and α1-adrenergic receptors are responsible for the side effects of sedation and orthostasis, similar to risperidone. Lastly, a comparative database analysis (of six double-blind, randomized, placebo-controlled, short term clinical trials) suggested that paliperidone ER dosed at 6.0-12.0 mg/day was more efficacious than risperidone 2.0-4.0 mg/day, and equally efficacious as risperidone 4.0-6.0 mg/day[86]. Interestingly, a placebo-adjusted adverse effect analysis revealed no difference in weight gain between these two medications. However, a case report in 2014 demonstrated a lower risk for weight gain and better appetite control after switching from risperidone (5.0 mg/day) to paliperidone (9.0 mg/day) in a patient with schizoaffective disorder[87]. Until additional randomized, head-to-head trials are published, the precise risk of metabolic adverse effects of paliperidone as compared to risperidone remain unknown.

ZIPRASIDONE

Ziprasidone appeared on the market in 2001 and is currently approved for both the acute and maintenance treatment of schizophrenia in adults, acute agitation in patients with schizophrenia, acute manic or mixed episodes of bipolar I disorder in adults (as monotherapy), and as maintenance therapy in bipolar I disorder (as adjunctive therapy to lithium or valproate)[88-90] (**Table 1**). Pharmacokinetically, ziprasidone clearly requires administration with food in order to maximize absorption and bioavailability (60.0% with food), and reaches peak plasma concentration in 6-8 hours[88] (**Table 4**). This drug requires a bi-daily dosing schedule given its shorter half-life and lower absorption. For the treatment of schizophrenia in adults, ziprasidone should be initiated at 20.0 mg twice daily, with subsequent dosage increases up to 80.0 mg twice daily[88] (**Table 1**). Dosing adjustments should occur in increments of 20.0 mg twice daily at intervals no less than 2 days, with a maximum dose of 80.0 mg twice daily. As with any SGA, patients should be observed prior to dosage increases, so as ensure the use of the lowest effective dose.

Although there is a paucity of evidence addressing the dosing strategy for the maintenance therapy of schizophrenia, a 44-week, randomized, double-blind, multicenter extension study demonstrated similar efficacy with either ziprasidone (80.0-160.0 mg/day) or risperidone (6.0-10.0 mg/day) in the treatment of patients with schizophrenia and schizoaffective disorder[91]. Although more subjects on ziprasidone failed to complete the study, there were fewer adverse effects (weight gain, EPS, and hyperprolactinemia) than the risperidone arm. In addition, a more recent report on the extension phase (3-73 month follow-up) of three multicenter, phase III studies, found ziprasidone to be well tolerated, with only mild to moderate adverse effects[92]. Lastly, the use of ziprasidone in schizophrenia is currently only approved for adults, and a recent placebo-controlled, long-term open extension study found no difference in efficacy between ziprasidone and placebo in the treatment of schizophrenia in adolescents (13-17 years)[93].

For the treatment of acute manic or mixed episodes of bipolar I disorder, an initial dose of 40.0 mg twice daily is recommended, with a dosage increase to 60.0-80.0 mg twice daily on the second day of treatment [88] (**Table 1**). If maintenance treatment is required (as an adjunct to lithium or valproate), patients can be maintained based on tolerability and efficacy within the range of 40.0-80.0 mg twice daily. Although not approved for the use in adolescents, a 4-week, randomized controlled trial (RCT) followed by a 26-week open-label extension study demonstrated ziprasidone (40.0-160.0 mg/day) was efficacious for the treatment of bipolar I disorder in children and adolescents (10-17 years)[94].

Interestingly, it has been shown that the use of the maximal FDA approved dose in patients with schizophrenia and bipolar disorder is associated with longer, sustained patient compliance[95]. This is most likely secondary to more efficacious symptom management and clinical effectiveness at higher doses (i.e. more D2 antagonism), therefore incentivizing patients to remain on the medication. In addition, it was observed that in state hospital systems the average dose of ziprasidone was 206 mg/day in the treatment of more refractory cases of schizophrenia and bipolar disorder[9]. Clinicians are therefore encouraged to ensure the use of maximal FDA approved doses of ziprasidone (unless safety or tolerability issues arise) before declaring treatment failure and turning to other treatment options. This clinical approach likely should be applied to all currently approved SGAs.

Currently, ziprasidone is not approved for the treatment of MDD or anxiety disorders, but there exists published studies suggesting potential antidepressant efficacy of this drug when compared to the limited data on risperidone or paliperidone[96]. An expert review suggested that similar to the FDA approved quetiapine, ziprasidone may be effective in mediating depressive and anxiety symptoms at low doses through pharamacodynamic mechanisms other than D2 antagonism[55,97]. Results of evidence-based clinical trials however have been inconsistent. Although large-scale studies have failed to demonstrate efficacy for the use in bipolar depression[98,99], smaller studies have suggested positive results[96,100-102]. For example, in an open-label trial of 20 failed responders with MDD, 61.5% achieved a response (and were classified as responders as measured by HAM-D-17 scores) after a 6-week trial of ziprasidone augmentation therapy[103]. However, a second 8-week open-label pilot study in 2007 found that although response rates were higher (and dose dependent) with ziprasidone augmentation (80.0 and 160.0 mg/day) as compared to sertraline monotherapy in patients with treatment resistant depression, there were no significant differences between groups[104]. These open-label trials also demonstrated good safety and tolerability, and may suggest some benefit of ziprasidone augmentation in patients with MDD. Further, in 2012, a 12-week randomized, placebo-controlled trial of ziprasidone monotherapy in patients with MDD found no significant differences in the reduction of depressive symptoms, response, or remission rates[98]. Of note however, a recently published randomized, double-blind, placebo-controlled 8-week trial of adjunctive ziprasidone demonstrated significant antidepressant efficacy (as measured by clinical response and HAM-D scores) in adults with MDD who had persistent symptoms after 8 weeks of open-label treatment with escitalopram[105]. Therefore, similar to risperidone, low-dose ziprasidone may exert some efficacy in the treatment of depressive and anxiety-related symptoms, while higher doses can be reserved for psychosis and mania.

As with all other SGAs, ziprasidone possesses the common strong D2/5-HT2a dual receptor antagonism responsible for its antipsychotic and antimanic properties[3,88,106] (**Table 5**). In regard to potential antidepressant effects, this drug also demonstrates strong 5-HT2c receptor antagonism, which similar to antagonism at the 5HT-2a receptor, results in an increased release of presynaptic dopamine and norepinephrine in the mesocortical pathway[3,26,107]. This action is believed to enhance concentration, attention, and executive functioning (i.e. the 'negative' symptoms of schizophrenia), with the exertion of these antidepressive effects at much lower doses than those necessary for the induction of antipsychotic properties (< 65.0% D2 receptor occupancy) via D2 blockade[1]. In addition, ziprasidone is a known agonist of 5-HT1a receptors that binds with high affinity (**Table 5**), similar to the action of the FDA approved anxiolytic buspirone, used in the treatment of GAD[108]. It is believed that the potential antidepressant effects of 5-HT1a agonists are mediated through postsynaptic receptors, while anxiolytic effects are mediated though presynaptic receptor modulation[109]. Lastly, ziprasidone demonstrates a relatively unique ability to inhibit both the norepinephrine and serotonin transporters (NET and SERT), similar to the mechanism of an SSRI/SNRI antidepressant[106].

Ziprasidone is characterized by relatively fewer adverse effects (as compared to some of the other SGAs), and is clinically described to have a lower risk of metabolic effects and weight gain[88]. Based upon the pharmacodynamic profile, ziprasidone binds with moderate affinity to histamine H1 receptors, high affinity to α1-adrenergic receptors, and little-to-no affinity to muscarinic M1 receptors[88] (**Table 5**). Therefore, clinicians should be aware of the potential for sedation, orthostatic hypotension, and dizziness associated with the use of this drug, especially with rapid dosing escalation. In addition, ziprasidone has been associated with prolongation of the QTc interval by 15.0-20.0 msec[88,110,111]. Although there were no noted cases of torsade de pointes during the pre-clinical trial program, patients may be monitored with both baseline and periodic EKGs if they have preexisting cardiac conditions. Along these lines, ziprasidone should be avoided or used judiciously in specific conditions: in combination with other drugs that prolong the QTc interval (class 1A and class III antiarrhythmics, certain antipsychotics, the fluoroquinolone antibiotics, pentamidine, methadone, and levomethadyl acetate); in patients with congenital prolongation of the QTc interval or a history of cardiac arrhythmias; recent acute myocardial infarction; and uncompensated heart failure[88]. It should also be noted that transient conditions such as hypokalemia, hypomagnesia, and bradycardia might also prolong the QTc interval, necessitating baseline and periodic electrolyte panels. Iloperidone is the only other SGA with similar precautions. Lastly, as ziprasidone is metabolized primarily by CYP3A4 (**Table 4**), the dose should be properly adjusted with the concomitant use of strong inhibitors or inducers of this enzyme, and the QTc interval monitored appropriately[88]. The enzyme CYP1A2 may contribute to the metabolism of ziprasdione to a much lesser extent[88], and therefore smoking (tobacco as a strong inducer of CYP1A2) should be cautioned with the use of this drug.

ILOPERIDONE

Iloperidone was approved by the FDA in 2009 and is currently only approved for the treatment of adults with schizophrenia[112-114] (**Table 1**). As the effectiveness of this drug has yet to be systematically evaluated in long-term randomized controlled trials, clinicians who elect to use iloperidone as maintenance therapy should periodically reassess for side effects and the need for long-term treatment. Although not randomized, placebo-controlled trials, three 52-week non-inferiority designed studies comparing iloperidone with haldoperidol in the treatment of adults with schizophrenia and schizoaffective disorder demonstrated similar relapse rates of these drugs, thus supporting a claim for maintenance efficacy in schizophrenia[115]. Oral bioavailability is 96.0% and time to peak plasma concentration is 2-4 hours[112] (**Table 4**). For dosing strategies, the recommended starting dose is 1.0 mg twice daily, with a target dose of 6.0-12.0 mg twice daily (12.0-24.0 mg/day) and maximum daily dose of 12.0 mg twice daily (24.0 mg/day)[112] (**Table 1**). Dosage increases and adjustments can be made daily at increments no greater than 2.0 mg twice daily (4.0 mg/day). This 'start low and go slow' titration strategy is due the very strong antagonism of α1-adrenergic receptors and subsequent risk for orthostatic hypotension (**Table 5**). Iloperidone generates two major metabolites, with the P88 metabolite able to cross the blood brain barrier, and possessing a pharmacodynamic profile equal or less to that of its parent compound[116]. Although metabolite P95 cannot cross the blood brain barrier, it has high affinity for both 5-HT2a and alpha-adrenergic receptors, which manifests clinically as a higher risk of postural hypotension[116].

In regard to off-label uses, MEDLINE and clinicaltrials. gov searches revealed minimal substantial clinical data for the use of iloperidone in the treatment of depression, anxiety, or bipolar disorder. Of note, a recently published 8-week placebo-controlled crossover study of iloperidone augmentation showed no significant improvements from placebo for residual anger and irritability in patients with partially remitted MDD[117]. In addition, a currently recruiting open-label, Phase 4 clinical trial plans to assess the efficacy of adjunct iloperidone (12.0-24.0 mg/day) therapy to ongoing adjustments can be made daily at treatment with lithium, divalproex, or lamotrigine in patients with bipolar disorder, mixed states[118].

Similar to other SGAs, iloperidone is proposed to exert its antipsychotic efficacy with lower risks of EPS through high affinity and antagonism of the D2 and 5-HT2a receptors[3,20,119] (**Table 5**). Although there is little clinical evidence for the use of iloperidone in the treatment of depression, its relative lack of 5-HT1a agonism, 5-HT2c antagonism, and serotonin/norepinephrine reuptake transporter (SERT/NET) inhibition suggests a pharmacodynamic profile more similar to that of risperidone, paliperidone, and olanzapine than that of quetiapine, ziprasidone, and asenapine (**Table 5**). Therefore, it could be reasonably assumed that a trial of low-dose iloperidone used as an augmentation strategy might demonstrate partial efficacy in patients with treatment resistant depression. In addition, iloperidone might exert antidepressant efficacy via a moderate affinity and antagonism of 5-HT7 receptors, similar to the previously discussed risperidone and paliperidone (these drugs however, demonstrate slightly higher 5-HT7 binding affinities than iloperidone; **Table 5**). Finally, iloperidone demonstrates moderate affinity and antagonism for 5-HT6 receptors, and evidence currently suggests that 5-HT6 antagonism may evoke antidepressant effects in animal models of MDD[55,120].

Pertaining to side effect profile, in addition to the atypical antipsychotic class effects described earlier (see risperidone), iloperidone use may have a higher incidence of orthostasis and dizziness due to its high affinity for the α1-adrenergic receptor (**Table 5**), and should therefore be used cautiously with antihypertensive agents. This drug demonstrates very low affinities for the histamine H1 and muscarinic M1-5 receptors, suggesting lower rates of sedation (**Table 5**). In addition, iloperidone has been noted to increase the cardiac QTc interval by ~9.0 msec at a dose of 12.0 mg twice daily[112,121]. Precautions similar to those previously described with the use of ziprasidone should be undertaken. Lastly, as iloperidone is a known substrate of both CYP2D6 and CYP3A4 (**Table 4**), the dose of iloperidone should be halved if there is concomitant use of strong inhibitors of these enzymes (i.e. fluoxetine and paroxetine for CYP2D6 and ketoconazole and clarithromycin for CYP3A4).

LURASIDONE

Lurasidone, one of the new SGAs, first appeared on the market in 2010 for the treatment of schizophrenia in adults, and was recently approved in 2013 for the treatment of depressive episodes associated with bipolar I in adults, either as monotherapy or adjunctive therapy to lithium or valproate[122] (**Table 1**). The effectiveness of this drug has yet to be systematically evaluated in long-term, randomized, placebo-controlled trials for either the treatment of schizophrenia or bipolar depression, and clinicians should therefore periodically reassess for adverse effects and the need for long-term treatment. However, a 12-month double-blind study in 2013 comparing lurasidone (40.0-160.0 mg/day) to quetiapine-ER (200.0-800.0 mg/day) demonstrated higher rates of remission and decreased risk of hospitalization with lurasidone[123]. Another long-term (12 month) double-blind, randomized, fixed dose study on the safety and tolerability of lurasidone (40.0-120.0 mg/day) as compared to risperidone (2.0-6.0 mg/day) found comparable efficacy between the two drugs, while lurasidone had greater rates of nausea, insomnia, sedation, and all-cause discontinuation[124]. Overall, the long-term use of lurasidone was well tolerated with minimal effects on metabolic outcomes. On the other hand, patients receiving risperidone experienced increased weight gain and serum prolactin levels (as compared to lurasidone).

The oral bioavailability of lurasidone is 9.0-19.0% with a peak plasma concentration of 1-3 hours (**Table 4**). Two separate food effect studies demonstrated an approximate 2-fold increase in oral bioavailability of lurasidone occurs when taken with meals (18.0-38.0%)[125]. It is therefore recommended that this drug be administered with food (at least 350 kcal) to ensure maximum exposure, similar to ziprasidone. Theoretically, doses may need to be doubled if taken without food.

Theoretically, doses may need to be doubled if taken without food. With respect to dosing strategies (**Table 1**), a starting dose of 40.0 mg/day (with no initial dose titration) is recommended for the treatment of adults with schizophrenia with an effective dosing range of 40.0-160.0 mg/day[122]. A lower starting dose of 20.0 mg/day is suggested for the treatment of depressive episodes associated with bipolar I disorder, with a therapeutic range of 20.0-120.0 mg/day[122]. A 6-week monotherapy trial however, demonstrated that higher doses (80.0-120.0 mg/day) not only failed to provide higher efficacy than lower dosages (20.0-60.0 mg/day), but was associated with increased side effect risk[126].

A MEDLINE and clinicaltrials.gov search regarding the off-label use of lurasidone for MDD revealed limited findings. A pooled analysis of short-term (6 weeks) placebo-controlled studies demonstrated lurasidone (40.0-160.0 mg/day) significantly improved depressive symptoms in patients with schizophrenia[127]. In addition, a recently completed (but yet to be published) 6-week, double-blind, placebo-controlled clinical trial (with a 12-week extension) was conducted to investigate the efficacy of low, flexibly-dosed lurasidone (20.0-60.0 mg/day) for the treatment of depressive disorder with mixed features[128,129]. Although preliminary, this trial suggests significant improvement in depressive symptoms, response rates, and remission rates as measured by the Montgomery-Asberg Depression Rating Scale (MADRS), the Clinical Global Impression-Severity of Illness (CGI-S) scores, the Young Mania Rating Scale (YMRS), the Sheehan Disability Scale (SDS), and the HAM-A. For the use of lurasidone for anxiety disorder, a MEDLINE and clinicaltrials.gov search revealed no clinical evidence.

As has been an ongoing theme for the SGAs, the antipsychotic properties and low EPS profile of high-dose lurasidone are most likely mediated through its very high affinity and dual antagonism of the D2/5-HT2a receptors[3,13,18](**Table

5). With respect to the antidepressant efficacy of lurasidone, the antagonism of 5-HT2a receptors in the mesocortical pathway and subsequent increased release of dopamine/norephinerphrine may improve concentration, attention, and executive functioning[3,13,25,27]. In addition, lurasidone is characterized by very strong antagonism of 5-HT7 receptors, moderate antagonism of α2A- and α2C-adrenergic receptors, and partial agonism of 5-HT1a receptors (**Table 5**), providing yet another potential mechanism for the mediation of depressive symptoms[13,76-79,85,109]. Therefore, based upon preliminary clinical evidence and pharmacodynamic profile, it remains feasible that lurasidone could be used as an efficacious augmentation therapy at lower dosages for the treatment of depressive symptoms in MDD.

Not accounting for the class effects of all SGAs (see risperidone), lurasidone has a relatively low side effect profile, as demonstrated by the very weak binding affinities for histamine H1 and muscarinic M1 receptors (**Table 5**). In addition, both lurasidone and ziprasidone have highly favorable metabolic profiles, with the lowest rates of metabolic adverse effects (weight gain, dyslipidemia, and diabetes risk) among the SGAs[130-139]. For example, a double-blind comparison trial of fixed-dose lurasidone (120.0 mg/day) demonstrated no clinically significant changes from baseline weight or metabolic parameters (total cholesterol and triglycerides)[133]. Interestingly, a six-month open label extension study provided evidence that switching from olanzapine (15.0 mg/day) to lurasidone (40.0-120.0 mg/day flexibly dosed) in schizophrenic patients was associated with significant weight loss and improved lipid/cardiometabolic parameters, while maintaining antipsychotic efficacy[137]. This decreased metabolic risk can perhaps be explained by the pharmacodynamic profile of lurasidone, which is characterized by low binding affinities for the histamine H1 and serotonergic 5-HT2c receptors (**Table 5**). Antagonism at these receptor sites has been previously implicated with increased metabolic risk[3,40-49].

As lurasidone is metabolized primarily by CYP3A4 (**Table 4**), the dose should be reduced to half with the concomitant use of strong CYP3A4 inhibitors (diltiazem, atazanavir, erythromycin, fluconazole, verapamil, ketoconazole, clarithromycin, ritonavir, voriconazole, and mibefradil). Grapefruit and grapefruit juice may inhibit CYP3A4, should therefore be avoided in patients taking lurasidone. The concomitant use of strong inducers of CYP3A4 (rifampin, avasimibe, St. John's wort, phenytoin, carbamazepine) should be avoided with lurasidone, and dosage increase may be necessary after chronic treatment (> 7 days) with moderate inducers.[122] Lastly, as lurasidone is not a substrate of CYP1A2, smoking should not have any effects on metabolism and pharmacokinetics of this drug.

CHAPTER 2

THE '-PINES'

OLANZAPINE

Olanzapine was first released on the market in 1996 and is currently approved for the treatment of schizophrenia in adults and adolescents, acute manic or mixed episodes associated with bipolar I disorder in adults and adolescents, the maintenance of bipolar I disorder in adults, and acute agitation associated with schizophrenia or bipolar disorder[140] (**Table 2**). In addition, a combination of olanzapine and fluoxetine is approved for the treatment of bipolar depression in both adults and adolescents, as well as treatment resistant MDD in adults[140] (**Table 2**). Olanzapine has an oral bioavailability of 87.0%[141], time to peak plasma concentration of 6 hours, a half life of 30 hours, and a time to steady state concentration of one week[140] (**Table 4**). This drug is extensively eliminated by first pass metabolism, with approximately 40.0% metabolized before reaching systemic circulation[140]. Food has little-to-no effect on the absorption of olanzapine.

Regarding dosing strategies, for the treatment of either schizophrenia or bipolar I mania (as monotherapy or adjunct to lithium or valproate), a target range of 10.0-15.0 mg/day with a maximum of 20.0 mg/day is recommend[140] (**Table 2**). As with other SGAs, adolescents are titrated to the same target range, but starting from lower doses. One study in 2009 suggested an average dose of 22.5 mg/day, with greater than 50% of patients above the recommended maximum dosage[10]. This study also discussed case reports in which patients received up to 60.0 mg/day with therapeutic efficacy. Interestingly, a small, follow-up prospective study demonstrated no improved efficacy and higher risks of weight gain and hyperprolactinemia associated with the use of higher doses (40.0 mg/day)[142]. A larger study also revealed no overall difference in efficacy between 20.0 and 40.0 mg/day, but did observe better responses to supra-therapeutic doses in patients with more severe baseline symptoms[143]. These studies suggest case by case management when prescribing supra-therapeutic doses of olanzapine; patients with more severe psychotic features may benefit from such off-label use, as there is a further increase in D2 receptor occupancy and antagonism to alleviate psychotic symptoms[1,3]. However, the use of such high doses is associated with a much greater risk of SGA side effects, and therefore full informed consent and increased drug monitoring should be practiced.

Although not indicated as monotherapy, low-dose olanzapine has nonetheless demonstrated at times antidepressant efficacy when used in such a treatment regiment[144-149]. When combined with fluoxetine however, olanzapine is more clearly effective and approved for the use in both bipolar depressive episodes and treatment resistant MDD[150-155]. As with other SGAs used in the treatment of depressive disorders, lower doses of olanzapine than needed for antipsychotic efficacy is recommended, typically starting at 3.0-6.0 mg/day, with a target range of 6.0-18.0 mg/day[140,145,156] (**Table 2**). Based on time to reach steady-state concentrations, medication adjustments should be spaced by one-week intervals, and patients monitored for treatment effectiveness and adverse events per usual. As discussed, the antidepressant efficacy of olanzapine at low doses is most likely mediated through its action on other receptor signaling pathways, and not via antagonism of the D2 receptors. There is very little literature to support the use of low-dose olanzapine in the treatment of anxiety disorders, either as adjunct or monotherapy[157-159], and larger, randomized, placebo-controlled trials are required to determine its anxiolytic efficacy.

Compared to risperidone and paliperidone, olanzapine has a slightly more complicated pharamacodynamic profile[140] (**Table 5**). Interestingly, the molecular structure of olanzapine is most similar to that of clozapine, a drug noted to be the most efficacious antipsychotic[140,160]. Olanzapine displays the characteristic D2 antagonism of most SGAs, but with only moderate binding affinities (**Table 5**). It also has the ability to antagonize 5-HT2a receptors with strong binding affinity, thereby decreasing the risks of EPS and hyperprolactinemia by allowing increased dopaminergic transmission in the nigrostriatal and tuberoinfundibular pathways, respectively[3,25-27]. Olanzapine's moderate affinity for 5-HT2c receptors may enhance dopamine and norepinerphrine activity in the mesocortical pathways, thereby contributing to its antidepressive efficacy[3,26,107]. For example, enhancement of signaling in the dorsolateral prefontal cortex may promote improved cognition, attention, concentration, and executive functioning, thereby providing treatment efficacy for not only the negative symptoms of schizophrenia, but also for symptoms of depression and anxiety. Olanzapine also demonstrates a moderate binding affinity for 5-HT6 receptors, providing another potential mechanism for its antidepressive efficacy[55,120]. There appears to be weak affinity for 5-HT7 and α2-adrenergic receptors, and little-to-no affinity for 5-HT1a receptors (**Table 5**).

Due to the moderate affinity and antagonism of the muscarinic M1 receptor (**Table 5**), olanzapine carries a greater risk of anticholinergic side effects than other SGAs, with the exception of perhaps quetiapine[140]. Patients should be monitored for constipation, urinary retention, dry mouth, sedation, blurred vision, and confusion. In addition, olanzapine is associated with a greater class effect risk of cardiomctabolic adverse events as compared to most other SGAs, including weight gain, hypertension, hyperlipidemia, and the development of type 2 diabetes mellitus[140]. Although it should be a practice implemented with the use of *all* SGAs, physicians are recommended to collect baseline and longitudinal screening data relevant to the development of these side effects (weight, waist circumference, blood pressure, lipid panel, glucose, and hemoglobin A1C). Olanzapine also demonstrates moderate and strong affinities for the α1-adrenergic and histamine H1 receptors, respectively, and patients should therefore be aware of the increased risks of dizziness, orthostatic hypotension, and sedation[140] (**Table 5**). Lastly, as olanzapine is a known substrate of both the CYP2D6 and CYP1A2 enzymes (**Table 4**), concomitant use with either inducers or inhibitors of these enzymes may necessitate olanzapine dosage increases or decreases, respectively[140].

QUETIAPINE

Released on the market in 1997, quetiapine was originally indicated for the treatment of both schizophrenia and bipiolar mania, similar to risperidone and olanzapine. In 2007, a slow-release (XR), once daily version of quetiapine was approved to improve patient compliance. Currently, this drug is approved for the treatment of schizophrenia and bipolar manic or mixed episodes in both adults and adolescents, the maintenance of bipolar I disorder in adults, acute depressive episodes associated with bipolar I disorder in adults, and as adjunctive therapy in adults with MDD[161] (**Table 2**). Quetiapine-XR has a time to peak plasma concentration of 6 hours and a time to reach steady-state concentration of 2 days[161] (**Table 4**). Due to extensive first pass metabolism, quetiapine is a SGA with a poor oral bioavailability of approximately 9.0%[162] (**Table 4**). In regard to dosing strategies, higher doses (400.0-800.0 mg/day) are required for antipsychotic and antimanic efficacy[161] (**Table 2**). Similar to olanzapine, although the adolescent target doses are the same as adults, a more conservative starting dose and titration strategy are implemented (**Table 2**). Interestingly, one study found that up to 40% of persistently ill patients in a New York State hospital system were being treated with more than 750.0 mg/day of quetiapine[11]. In addition, anecdotal reports indicate the efficacious use of this drug at doses above 800.0 mg/day, and even up to 2400.0 mg/day[12].

With respect to the treatment of bipolar I depression and as adjunctive therapy for MDD in adults, the use of low-dose quetiapine has demonstrated antidepressive efficacy in multiple, randomized, placebo-controlled trials[163-168]. For example, 400.0-600.0 mg/day is recommended for the treatment of bipolar depression as monotherapy, and 150.0-300.0 mg/day of quetiapine as adjunct to SSRI or SNRI antidepressants[161] (**Table 2**). Although not indicted for use as monotherapy in adults with

MDD, four out of five acute studies have demonstrated that low-dose quetiapine-XR monotherapy improved depressive symptoms in patients with MDD, as compared to placebo[169-172]. The fifth study demonstrated no improvement (as compared to placebo) for either quetiapine-XR or escitalopram monotherapy in patients with MDD[173]. In addition, although similarly not approved for the treatment of anxiety disorders, a recent review of literature[174] and meta-analysis of randomized controlled trials[175] suggested low-dose quetiapine-XR (50.0-150.0 mg/day) as an efficacious off-label treatment option in adults with GAD who had failed to respond to conventional antidepressant therapy. The review of literature assessed data from trials using quetiapine as either monotherapy or adjunct therapy, while the meta-analysis focused only on randomized controlled trials using quetiapine-XR as monotherapy. The use of such low doses to treat depression and anxiety most likely does not require antagonism of dopamine transmission to the extent observed with higher, antipsychotic doses. As discussed below, the antidepressive and anxiolytic efficacy of quetiapine is therefore a product of its action on other receptor signaling pathways.

As assessed by its pharmacodynamic profile, quetiapine is considered to be a low potency, or low affinity drug, due to weak binding affinities to and antagonism of D2 receptors (**Table 5**). Although this doesn't translate to a drug of low effectiveness, it does suggest that quetiapine requires higher doses (400.0-800.0 mg/day) to maintain the necessary 65.0% D2 receptor occupancy for antipsychotic and antimanic efficacy[1,161]. In addition, this weak D2 binding affinity may allow for a decreased risk of EPS[3]. Quetiapine also demonstrates moderate antagonism of 5-HT2a receptors (**Table 5**), which not only lowers EPS rates but also improves cognition and the negative symptoms of schizophrenia, as previously discussed for other SGAs[3,25-27]. There also appears to be weak affinity for and antagonism of both 5-HT7 and α2-adrenergic receptors, which may mediate some of the antidepressive and anxiolytic efficacy of this drug at low doses[76-78]. To complicate matters, the main active metabolite, norquetiapine, demonstrates a unique pharmacodynamic profile from that of its parent drug[161] (**Table 5**). More specifically, norquetiapine has a greater affinity for 5-HT2a and 5-HT7 receptors than quetiapine, and adds a weak antagonism of 5-HT2c and 5-HT6 receptors. These antagonistic properties are believed to foster pro-cognitive and antidepressive effects[3,26,55,79,120]. There appears to be a similar weak D2/D3 antagonism for both norquetiapine and its parent drug. Interestingly, norquetiapine also demonstrates two unique pharmacodynamic features. The first is a weak 5-HT1a partial agonism, which as previously discussed demonstrates anxiolytic efficacy in a similar manner to buspirone[108,109]. Second, the metabolite norquetiapine is a moderate inhibitor of the NET (**Table 5**), acting in a similar manner as the FDA approved antidepressants venlafaxine, duloxetine, buproprion, nortryptiline, and desipramine[3,161]. This relatively unique property (shared only with ziprasidone) most likely improves cognition, energy, concentration, depression, and anxiety in a clinical setting similar to the aforementioned FDA approved antidepressants. Again, although the use of low-dose quetiapine demonstrates less antipsychotic and antimanic efficacy (due to decreased D2 antagonism), its serotonergic and noradrenergic pharmacodynamic properties at such doses are believed to be largely responsible for the amelioration of depressive and anxiety-related symptoms.

As both quetiapine and norquetiapine are characterized by strong histamine H1 receptor antagonism, clinicians should be aware of the increased risk of sedation and cardiometabolic side effects[161] (**Table 5**). Although H1 antagonism is often associated with fatigue and somnolence and may lead to poor patient compliance, these adverse events may be used to improve insomnia or agitation, similar to other antihistamines[3]. Quetiapine demonstrates little-to-no antagonism of muscarinic M1 receptors, and therefore has a relatively low anticholinergic side effect risk[161] (**Table 5**). However, norquetiapine has a moderate affinity for M1 receptors comparable to that of olanzapine, thus increasing the risk of such adverse events. Lastly, both quetiapine and its metabolite demonstrate moderate affinity for α1-adrenergic receptors, and patients should be cautioned and monitored for the increased risks of dizziness and orthostatic hypotension. As previously mentioned, quetiapine is associated with a high first-pass metabolism and is largely metabolized by the CYP3A4 enzyme[161] (**Table 4**). Therefore, the concomitant use of inducers (phenytoin, carbamazepine, rifampin, St. John's wort) or inhibitors (ketoconazole, itraconazole, indinavir, ritonavir, nefazodone) of CYP3A4 requires a 5-fold increase and one-sixth reduction of the original quetiapine dose[161].

ASENAPINE

In 2009, asenapine was simultaneously approved for the treatment of adults with schizophrenia and bipolar mania[176] (**Table 2**). The oral bioavailability is approximately 35.0% and the drug reaches peak plasma concentrations within 0.5-1.5 hours and has a half life of 24 hours[176] (**Table 4**). Asenapine tablets must be taken sublingually (no splitting, crushing, chewing, or swallowing) and without the intake of food or drink up to 15 minutes after administration to ensure proper absorption. Dosing in schizophrenia is typically initiated and maintained at 5.0 mg twice daily with a maximum daily dose of 10.0 mg twice daily[176] (**Table 2**). If titration is necessary, the starting dose can be increased up to 10.0 mg twice daily after one week. In the treatment of adults with manic or mixed episodes secondary to bipolar I disorder, asenapine can be started at 10.0 mg twice daily as either a monotherapy or as adjunctive treatment to lithium or valproate[176]. The dose can be subsequently decreased to 5.0 mg twice daily in the advent of adverse side effects. Lastly, in 2015 asenapine was approved as monotherapy for the treatment of adolescents (10-17 years) with acute manic or mixed bipolar I episodes[176]. In this population, dosing is initiated at 2.5 mg twice daily, and can be increased to 5.0 mg twice daily on day 3 and 10 mg twice daily on day 6 if needed (**Table 2**).

Although initially approved based on short-term trials[176], more recent studies investigating the long-term use of asenapine for treatment of adults with schizophrenia[177-180] and bipolar disorder[181] have demonstrated efficacy, safety, and tolerability. In particular, one study found asenapine (5.0-10.0 mg twice daily) to be superior to olanzapine (5.0-20.0 mg/day) in regard to improving the negative symptoms associated with schizophrenia with continued treatment up to 52 weeks[177]. Another trial suggested that although asenapine was well tolerated at 1 year of treatment, there was less weight gain and greater EPS risk as compared to olanzapine[178]. However, an extension of this study (up to 3 years treatment) found similar clinical stability between both drugs, with negligible adverse effects beyond 1 year[179].

Regarding the effectiveness of asenapine in the treatment of MDD, although a MEDLINE search reviewed no published trials, a clinicaltrials.gov search identified two relevant studies. The first was a Phase 2 trial comparing asenapine to placebo in the treatment of bipolar depression over 8 weeks, and is currently recruiting[182]. The second was a 6-week, Phase 4 trial of asenapine augmentation to antidepressant therapy in patients with MDD who have yet to respond to antidepressant therapy alone[183]. This trial was completed with results, but has yet to be published. A MEDLINE and clinicaltrials.gov search for the use of asenapine in the treatment of anxiety disorders found no current clinical evidence, with the exception of a single animal study suggesting asenapine may have anxiolytic-like properties in mice[184].

Similar to other SGAs, asenapine demonstrates antipsychotic and antimanic efficacy with lowered risks of EPS due to its dual D2/5-HT2a blockade[3,21,22,185]. In fact, asenapine demonstrates one of the highest binding affinities to 5-HT2a receptors (**Table 5**), thereby providing a potential mechanism for its efficacy in the treatment of the negative symptoms of schizophrenia[3,25-27], and possibly depression/anxiety. Interestingly, this drug shares a similar molecular structure with the antidepressant mirtazapine[176] and is believed to enhance both serotonin and norepinephrine activity in the cortex[186]. In addition to the mesocortical antagonism of 5-HT2a receptors, the pharmacodynamic profile of asenapine suggests some treatment possibilities in patients with depression and anxiety (**Table 5**). Specifically, this drug demonstrates strong partial agonism of 5-HT1a receptors, very strong antagonism of 5-HT2b/c, 5-HT6, and 5-HT7 receptors, and strong to very strong antagonism of the α2A/B/C-adrenergic receptors, which in turn mediate pro-cognitive and antidepressive effects[21,22,55,76-79,85,109,120,176]. Similar to the previously discussed SGAs, these potential antidepressive effects are most likely mediated at lower doses than needed for antipsychotic efficacy.

The pharmacodyanmic profile of asenapine also demonstrates high affinity for histamine H1 and α1-adrenergic receptor antagonism[176] (**Table 5**), and clinicians should therefore be aware of the potential for sedation, orthostatic hypotension, and dizziness associated with this drug, in addition to the previously discussed class effects (see risperidone). Asenapine demonstrates little-to-no affinity for muscarinic M1 receptors, and therefore has a very low risk of anticholinergic side effects. In addition, caution should be exercised when asenapine is used in patients taking antihypertensive agents, as asenapine may enhance the effects of these drugs[176]. Patients should undergo periodic blood pressure monitoring and the dosage of the antihypertensive drug adjusted accordingly. Asenapine is primarily metabolized by UGT1A4 (direct glucuronidation) and CYP1A2, and to a lesser extent, CYP3A4 and CYP2D6[176]. Co-administration of strong inhibitors (fluvoxamine, ciprofloxacin, and verapamil) or inducers (tobacco, i.e. smoking) of CYP1A2 would therefore necessitate either asenapine dosage adjustments (decreases or increases, respectively) based on clinical response. It is also known that asenapine is itself a weak inhibitor CYP2D6, and may enhance the inhibitory effects of SSRIs such as fluoxetine and paroxetine on their own metabolism[176]. Indeed, as the concomitant use of asenapine and paroxetine increased paroxetine exposure by 2-fold[176], a reduction of the paroxetine dosage by half is recommended when these two drugs are administered in combination.

CHAPTER 3

THE '-PIPS' AND '-RIPS'

ARIPIPRAZOLE

Aripiprazole was first released in 2002, approved solely for the acute and maintenance treatment of schizophrenia. As of 2016 however, aripiprazole has achieved a wide range of approvals, including the management of acute agitation associated with schizophrenia and bipolar I disorder, the acute and maintenance treatment of manic or mixed episodes in bipolar I disorder (both adults and adolescents), irritability and aggression associated with autism, Tourette's disorder, and as adjunct treatment for MDD[187] (**Table 3**). Aripiprazole has an oral bioavailability of 87.0% and time to peak plasma concentration of 3 to 5 hours[187] (**Table 4**). This drug is associated with a very long half-life and time to steady-state concentration of 75 hours and 14 days, respectively (**Table 4**), and can be taken with or without food. As a consequence of the long time to reach steady-state levels, dosage adjustments should be made at intervals no less than one week and patients monitored for efficacy and adverse effects. For the treatment of psychosis associated with schizophrenia, a starting and target dose of 10.0 or 15.0 mg/day is recommended, up to a maximum of 30.0 mg/day[187] (**Table 3**). Dosing adjustments should occur at 5.0 mg increments at intervals no sooner than two weeks (i.e. the time needed to achieve state-state concentrations). As with other SGAs, adolescent dosing is more conservative, with a recommended starting dose of 2.0 mg/day, and titrations to 5.0 mg on day 2 and 10.0 mg on day 4[187] (**Table 3**). Dosing strategies in acute manic or mixed episodes secondary to bipolar I disorder in both adults and adolescents are similar to those discussed for schizophrenia. For adjunctive treatment of MDD, aripiprazole is used in lowered doses, with a starting dose of 2.0-5.0 mg/day and target range of 2.0-15.0 mg/day. Adjustments should be made at 5.0 mg increments at intervals no less than one week (**Table 3**).

Interestingly, despite its later market release, aripiprazole was the first FDA approved drug to be used as an augmentation strategy in MDD, whereas quetiapine-XR was approved later. The efficacy of adjunctive aripiparzole in MDD has been demonstrated not only through numerous small-scale open studies[188-193], but also in both short and long-term (up to 52 weeks) randomized, placebo-controlled trials[194-199]. In some of these studies, remission was achieved within one or two weeks of augmentation therapy[194,195]. The randomized, placebo-controlled trials also demonstrated that aripiprazole augmentation was safe and well tolerated, with completion and discontinuation rates similar to placebo (85.0% vs. 87.0% and 4.4% vs. 1.7%, respectively)[55]. The most common side effects were mild-to-moderate akathisia (23.0% of patients) and significant weight gain. These adverse events were similar to those observed in long-term studies, which reported higher rates for akathisia, weight gain, and fatigue as compared to placebo[199]. At the lower doses used to treat MDD (2.0-15.0 mg/day), the reduction in dopamine transmission which mediates antipsychotic/antimanic efficacy is not required. Instead, low-dose aripiprazole (similar to other SGAs) promotes dopamine, norepinephrine, and serotonin transmission through complex interactions with a variety of receptor signaling pathways to mediate these antidepressive and anxiolytic effects.

In discussing the off-label use of aripiprazole to treat anxiety disorders, there are published small, open-label trials demonstrating efficacy in the treatment of GAD and PD with low doses of aripiprazole (13.9 mg/day)[200,201]. Interestingly, the use of high-dose aripiprazole (up to 30.0 mg/day) for up to 12 months in patients with schizophrenia and co-occurring social anxiety demonstrated improved social anxiety, psychosis, and quality of life, with improvements observed within the first 8 weeks of treatment[202]. Animal models have also suggested this drug can inhibit anxiety-related responses and alleviate aversive states, even those induced by ethanol[203,204]. These anxiolytic effects are perhaps mediated through aripiprazole's strong affinity for (and partial agonism of) 5-HT1a receptors, similar to the mechanism of action for buspirone, an FDA approved anxiolytic[108,109]. Lastly, although not classified as an anxiety disorder by the DSM-5, aripiprazole is currently approved for the treatment of irritability associated with autism and Tourette's disorder[187]. In addition, a clinicaltrials.gov search revealed two completed trials (with no associated publications) in regard to the use of aripiprazole for the treatment of post-traumatic stress disorder[205] and schizophrenia with symptoms of obsessive-compulsive disorder[206]. Only a single clinical trial (completed with no associated publications) was found investigating the efficacy of low-dose aripiprazole for 8 weeks in refractory anxiety[207].

With the previously discussed SGAs, antipsychotic efficacy is achieved primarily via antagonism of D2 receptors[1,3]. Aripiprazole however has a unique pharmacodynamic profile in that it binds with very high affinity to D2 receptors, but acts as a strong partial *agonist* at this receptor, instead of the classically described SGA D2 full antagonist[187] (**Table 5**). Aripiprazole can therefore be considered an *atypical* atypical, or third generation antipsychotic (TGA), and this unique mechanism of action is shared by the two other drugs in this class (brexpiprazole and cariprazine). Partial agonism suggests a balancing act between the partial stimulation of D2 receptors in areas of *hypo*dopaminergic activity (mesocortical pathway) and the partial dampening of endogenous dopamine in areas of *hyper*dopaminergic activity (mesolimbic pathway) to mediate antipsychotic efficacy[23,187,208-213]. The discovery of D2 partial agonists has therefore allowed for the development of a well-tolerated treatment with stabilizing effects on dopamine function in multiple brain pathways, all mediated through a single receptor. However, similar to all SGAs, aripiprazole has a complex pharmacodynamic profile, and the additional targets may broaden clinical treatment opportunities and may even generate unintentional side effects. In addition, aripiprazole demonstrates a high affinity for and strong partial agonism of the D3 receptor[187] (**Table 5**). Although partial agonism of this receptor may not lend itself to antipsychotic efficacy, it is proposed to promote dopaminergic activity in cortical areas, thereby exerting potential pro-cognitive, alertness, and antidepressive effects[3,208,209]. Lastly, aripiprazole demonstrates high to very high affinity to and antagonism of 5-HT2a/b/c receptors, moderate affinity to 5-HT7 receptors, and acts as a strong partial agonist of 5-HT1a receptors (**Table 5**), which as previously discussed, diminishes EPS risks and promotes cognition and antidepressant potential[25-27,55,78,109,187]. Aripiprazole also demonstrates weak inhibition of the SERT, similar to the mechanism of SSRIs[23,187] (**Table 5**).

As aripiprazole demonstrates moderate affinity and antagonism of both the histamine H1 and α1-andrenergic receptors (**Table 5**), clinicians should be aware of the possible adverse events of sedation, dizziness, and orthostatic hypotension[187]. In addition, aripiprazole appears to be associated with a higher risk of akathisia (perhaps due to its very high affinity for D2 receptors), as compared to other SGAs[187]. Clinically, aripiprazole has a lower risk of weight gain and metabolic-related side effects as compared to risperidone, olanzapine, and quetiapine. Relating to metabolism, aripiprazole is a known substrate of both CYP3A4 and CYP2D6 enzymes (**Table 4**). Its major metabolite, dehydro-aripiprazole, has similar affinities for D2 receptors as its parent drug, with a half-life of 94 hours and time to steady-state concentration of two weeks[187]. Therefore, daily dosing should be halved in patients simultaneously taking strong inhibitors of either CYP2D6 or CYP3A4. In addition, physicians should proceed cautiously in patients known to be CYP2D6 poor metabolizers or with the concomitant use of aripiprazole and strong inducers of either CYP2D6 or CYP3A4, regularly monitoring their patients for both clinical efficacy and adverse events related to aberrant metabolism.

BREXPIPRAZOLE

Brexpiprazole is one of the newest SGAs, approved (July 2015) for the treatment of schizophrenia and as adjunctive therapy to MDD in adults[214] (**Table 3**). It has a high oral bioavailability of 95.0% and reaches peak plasma concentrations within 4 hours[214] (**Table 4**). Interestingly, brexpiprazole has a half-life of 91 hours and time to steady state concentration of 10-12 days, much longer than most of the previously discussed SGAs (**Table 4**). For the treatment of schizophrenia, the recommended starting dose is 1.0 mg/day with a target dosage of 2.0-4.0 mg/day and a maximum of 4.0 mg/day[214] (**Table 3**). If dose titration is needed, an increase to 2.0 mg/day on day 4 and 4.0 mg/day on day 8 is recommended. When using brexpiprazole as an adjunct treatment to MDD in adults, patients can be started on a lower dose of 0.5-1.0 mg/day with titrations up to 1.0 or 2.0 mg/day at weekly intervals, and a maximum of 3.0 mg/day[214].

Although two distinct 6-week randomized, double-blind, placebo-controlled trials demonstrated the efficacy of brexpiprazole in the acute management of adults with schizophrenia[214], a MEDLINE search revealed no current publications with respect to the long-term or maintenance treatment of schizophrenia with this drug. A clinicaltrials.gov search found two Phase 3 studies investigating the efficacy, safety, and tolerability of brexpiprazole in the maintenance (up to 52 weeks) of adults with schizophrenia[215,216]. Lastly, there is an actively recruiting Phase 1 trial with plans to assess the safety and tolerability of brexpiprazole in adolescents with schizophrenia[217]. Both a MEDLINE and clinicaltrials.gov search found no currently published or ongoing investigations into the use of brexpiprazole as monotherapy for the treatment of MDD. Lastly, due to the recent FDA approval of this drug, a MEDLINE and clinicaltrials.gov search revealed no clinical evidence for the use of brexpiprazole in the treatment of anxiety or bipolar disorders.

The pharmacodynamic profile of brexpiprazole is similar to that of the previously discussed aripiprazole, demonstrating antipsychotic efficacy through a strong partial *agonism* at the D2 receptor[15,214] (**Table 5**). The partial agonism results in both increased dopamine signaling in areas of *hypo*dopaminergic activity (mesocortical pathway) and a reduction of endogenous dopamine signaling in areas of *hyper*dopaminergic activity (mesolimbic pathway) to exert antipsychotic efficacy[14,15,23,208-211,218,219]. This partial agonism also decreases the risk of EPS and hyperprolactinemia (as compared to complete D2 antagonists), as mediated by a less prominent decrease of the endogenous dopamine signaling in the nigrostriatal and tuberoinfundibular pathways, respectively. In addition, brexipiprazole demonstrates a high affinity for and strong partial agonism of the D3 receptor[15,214] (**Table 5**), and similar to aripiprazole, is believed to exert potential pro-cognitive and antidepressive effects[3,208,209]. Lastly, brexpiprazole demonstrates high to very high affinity for and antagonism of α2-adrenergic, 5-HT2a/b, and 5-HT7 receptors and acts as a partial agonist of 5-HT1a receptors (**Table 5**), which as previously discussed, diminishes EPS risks and promotes cognition and antidepressant potential[55,76-79,85,109,214]. Interestingly, as compared to aripiprazole, brexpiprazole has demonstrated both a lower intrinsic activity at D2 receptors and higher binding affinities for 5-HT1a/2a receptors[15,214] (**Table 5**). This suggests brexpiprazole might have a favorable antipsychotic potential with a decreased incidence of side effects (especially akathisia) related to D2 receptor partial agonism.

In double-blind trials for the treatment of acute schizophrenia, discontinuation rates were lower for patients receiving brexpiprazole (2.0-4.0 mg/day) as compared to placebo (7.0% vs. 9.0%)[23,220,221]. Interestingly, in acute MDD trials in which brexpiprazole was prescribed at lower doses, there was a higher rate of discontinuation secondary to adverse events in those receiving brexpiprazole as compared to placebo (3.0% vs. 1.0%), yielding a number needed to harm (NNH) of 50[23,222,223]. The most commonly observed adverse events in trials investigating the use of brexpiprazole as adjunctive treatment in MDD were akathisia (8.6% vs. 1.7%; NNH 15) and weight gain (6.7% vs. 1.9%; NNH 22)[23,214]. The rate of akathisia was also observed to be dose-related. The most commonly observed adverse event in the treatment of schizophrenia was weight gain (4.0% vs. 2.0%), with a NNH of 50[23,214]. It is important to note that in schizophrenia trials, there was no significant difference in the rate of akathisia between brexpiprazole and placebo (5.5% vs. 4.6%; NNH 112)[214]. The effects on glucose and lipids in these trials were negligible. With respect to aripiprazole, the most commonly encountered adverse event was akathisia, whether it was used to treat schizophrenia (8.0% vs. 4.0%; NNH 25), bipolar mania as monotherapy (13.0% vs. 4.0%; NNH 12), bipolar mania as adjunct (19.0 vs. 5.0%; NNH 8), or MDD as adjunct (25.0% vs. 4.0%; NNH 5)[23,187]. In addition, a 6-week exploration study revealed the incidence of EPS-related events (akathisia) were lower in patients treated with brexpiprazole, as compared to aripiprazole (14.1% vs. 30.3%), yielding a non-significant number needed to treat (NNT) of 7 in the advantage of brexpiprazole[224].

Overall, it would appear that the adverse events associated with these partial D2 agonists (weight gain, akathisia, and somnolence) are more frequently observed when used for the indication of mood disorders as compared to schizophrenia (as assessed by NNH), with akathisia being the most frequent of these events[23]. When broken down by rank order of propensity for the indication of schizophrenia, the risk for weight gain is greatest in brexpiprazole, followed by aripiprazole, and finally cariprazine[23]. The risk for akathisia on the other hand (when used for the indication of schizophrenia) is greatest for cariprazine, followed by aripiprazole, and lowest for brexpiprazole. These rank orders however were based upon an indirect comparison of NNH and properly designed head-to-head studies are required to accurately elucidate potential differences in adverse events. In addition, it is important to note that these adverse events are based primarily upon acute studies and therefore cannot be used to comment on adverse events such as tardive dyskinesia, long-term weight gain, or the development of type 2 diabetes mellitus, all of which require time to manifest.

As brexpiprazole binds with moderate affinity to histamine H1 receptors and strong to very strong affinity to α1-adrenergic receptors (**Table 5**), physicians should be aware of the potential risk for sedation, dizziness, and orthostatic hypotension with the use of this drug (in addition to the class effect risk of all SGAs)[214]. Brexpiprazole has little-to-no binding affinity for the muscarinic M1 receptor. Metabolism of brexpiprazole is mediated primarily by the CYP3A4 and CYP2D6 enzymes[214] (**Table 4**). Its major metabolite, DM-3411, is not believed to play a role in the therapeutic effects of this drug, and there is little to no inhibition of the CYP450 isoenzymes with its use[214]. Therefore, in patients classified as CYP2D6 poor metabolizers and in those prescribed strong CYP2D6 or CYP3A4 inhibitors, brexpiprazole should be titrated to half of the usual dose. Genetic polymorphisms account for the phenotypic variability of the CYP2D6 isoenzyme (ranging from poor to ultrarapid metabolizers), with differences in prevalence among ethnicities[225-227]. On the other hand, the concomitant use of brexpiprazole and strong inducers of CYP3A4 requires a doubling of the usual dose over 1 to 2 weeks. Lastly, a quarter of the usual dose of brexpiprazole is recommended with either the administration of strong CYP3A4 inhibitors in CYP2D6 poor metabolizers, or the co-administration of strong to moderate CYP2D6 and CYP3A4 inhibitors.

CARIPRAZINE

As the most novel addition to the SGAs (September 2015), cariprazine is currently approved for the treatment of adults with schizophrenia and as monotherapy for manic or mixed episodes associated with bipolar I disorder[228] (**Table 3**). This drug is characterized by a high oral bioavailability, reaching 52.0% in rats dosed with 1.0 mg/kg, and due to its lipophilic properties, can easily cross the blood brain barrier[228]. Cariprazine has the longest SGA half-life (2-4 days) and time to steady state concentration (1-2 weeks), although it reaches peak plasma concentration within 3-6 hours[228] (**Table 4**). Interestingly, one of the two major active metabolites of cariprazine, didesmethyl cariprazine (DDCAR) approaches steady state concentrations around 4-8 weeks, with a half-life between 1-3 weeks[228]. Due to these unique pharamacokinetic properties, dosage changes will not be reflected in plasma concentration for weeks, and clinicians are therefore recommended to monitor for therapeutic response and adverse effects for several weeks after initiation and dosage adjustments. These long half-lives are most common within the '-pip/-rip' family.

In adults with schizophrenia, the recommended starting dose is 1.5 mg/day[228] (**Table 3**). If needed, the dose can be increased to 3.0 mg/day on day 2, with further adjustments made in either 1.5 mg or 3.0 mg increments at several week intervals (as determined by the aforementioned long half-life). This same dosing strategy is also used in adults with manic or mixed episodes secondary to bipolar I disorder. Although cariprazine has demonstrated clinical efficacy up to 9.0 mg/day for the treatment of schizophrenia[229] and up to 12.0 mg/day in bipolar I disorder[230-232], the effectiveness of dosages above 6.0 mg/day was not sufficient to outweigh dose-related side effects, and the recommended maximum dose is therefore 6.0 mg/day[228] (**Table 3**).

A MEDLINE and clinicaltrials.gov search revealed no published studies for to the use of cariprazine in the treatment of schizophrenia in adolescents. Regarding the long-term use of cariprazine as maintenance therapy in schizophrenia, only three completed clinical trials (with no associated publications) were found. The first was a randomized, double-blind, placebo-controlled trial investigating the prevention of relapse in patients with schizophrenia treated with long-term (up to 92 weeks), flexibly-dosed (3.0-9.0 mg/day) cariprazine[233]. The other two studies sought to determine the safety, tolerability, and pharmacokinetics of cariprazine when administered up to 48 weeks[234,235]. The efficacy of cariprazine was established in the acute treatment of bipolar mania in three distinct, 3-week, placebo-controlled trials[228,230-232]. In regard to long-term management (either as monotherapy or adjunct), a MEDLINE and clinicaltrials. gov search revealed only a single completed, 16-week, open-label, Phase 3 trial (with no associated publications) investigating the long-term tolerability of cariprazine monotherapy in patients with bipolar I disorder[236].

With respect to the off-label use of cariprazine, a recently published, 8-week, randomized, double-blind, placebo-controlled study demonstrated efficacy (as assessed by improvements in MADRS and CGI-S) of low-dose cariprazine monotherapy (1.5 mg/day) for the treatment of bipolar I depression [237]. The treatment was well tolerated; the most common side effects observed were akathisia and insomnia, with weight gain slightly higher in the cariprazine groups. A rat model of chronic mild stress also suggested cariprazine had antidepressant effects with greater potency than aripiprazole[238]. A clinicaltrials.gov search revealed five completed trials (with no associated publications) and a single actively recruiting trial investigating the use of cariprazine as either monotherapy[239,240] or adjunctive therapy[241-244] for the treatment of MDD. Both a MEDLINE and clinicaltrials.gov search revealed no clinical evidence for the use of cariprazine in the treatment of

anxiety disorders. Although there is very little published evidence
for the use of cariprazine in MDD, the aforementioned trials
and unique pharamacodynamic profile of this drug suggest that
cariprazine may demonstrate antidepressive efficacy at doses lower
than those used to ameliorate psychotic or manic symptoms.

Similar to aripiprazole and brexpiprazole, the
pharmacodynamic profile of cariprazine reveals partial *agonism*
of D2 and D3 receptors[16,228] (**Table 5**). Although these three drugs
have similar binding affinities for the D2 receptor (Ki < 1.0),
cariprazine demonstrates a much greater affinity for D3 receptors
(Ki < 0.1) as compared to aripiprazole and brexpiprazole (1.0 <
Ki > 0.1;**Table 5**). As previously discussed (see aripiprazole and
brexpiprazole), this strong partial agonism of D2/D3 receptors
is thought to mediate the antipsychotic and antimanic effects of
cariprazine at high doses[23,208-211,245]. Interestingly, cariprazine binds
with only moderate affinity as an antagonist of 5-HT2a receptors,
as compared to most other SGAs (with the exception of quetiapine),
which bind with high affinities (**Table 5**). This observation,
coupled with a low binding affinity to 5-HT2c receptors[228],
would presumably put cariprazine at higher risks of EPS and
hyperprolactinemia, as these adverse effects are believed to be
countered via antagonism at these receptors in the nigrostriatal and
tuberoinfundibular pathways, respectively[3]. Indeed, some of the
most common side effects observed in clinical trials with high-dose
cariprazine were EPS and akathisia, with lower rates of dyspepsia,
vomiting, and somnolence[23,228]. However, the unique D2/D3
partial agonism may curb some of this risk, lowering the levels of
endogenous dopamine activity in these areas to a lesser extent than
a full antagonist. This partial agonism of D2/D3 receptors may
account for the potential antidepressive and pro-cognitive effects of
cariprazine, though attenuation of the hyperdopaminergic activity
in the mesocortical pathway[3,208,209]. In addition, cariprazine
acts as a partial agonist at 5-HT1a receptors and antagonist of
5-HT2b receptors, binding with high and very high affinity,

respectively[228] (**Table 5**). There is also observed moderate-to-weak binding and antagonism of 5-HT7 receptors and little-to-no binding to α2-adrengeric receptors[228]. As previously discussed, modulation of these receptors has been linked to antidepressant and pro-cognitive efficacy[3,25-27,78,109].

Cariprazine binds to the histamine H1 receptor with high-to-moderate affinity[16,228] (**Table 5**), thereby increasing the risk of somnolence and sedation at higher and more rapidly titrated doses, as was observed in clinical trials[23,228]. Interestingly, as compared to other SGAs (**Table 5**), cariprazine binds with low affinity to α1-adrenergic receptors, suggesting a lower risk of orthostatic hypotension and dizziness, although these adverse effects should not be dismissed. As discussed above, this drug appears to carry a slightly higher risk of EPS, perhaps due to a decreased antagonism of 5-HT2a/c receptors combined with a very high affinity for D2 receptors[23,228]. As with all SGAs, clinicians should be aware of class effects common to this class of drugs (see risperidone). In regard to elimination, cariprazine is metabolized primarily by CYP3A4 to desmethyl cariprazine (DCAR) and didesmethyl cariprazine (DDCAR), both of which are pharmacologically equipotent and demonstrate similar receptor binding profiles to their parent drug[228]. Similar to their parent drug, these two metabolites demonstrate extremely long half-lives and times to reach steady state concentrations. Caution and proper dosage adjustments are recommended in patients with the concomitant use of cariprazine and strong CYP3A4 inducers and inhibitors.

DISCUSSION

As a generalization, all SGAs have the necessary pharmacological properties to ameliorate psychosis and mania when used near their highest dosing ranges. This efficacy is primarily due to optimal levels of dopamine D2 receptor blockade and antagonism in the mesolimbic pathway, but at such high doses there is a greater risk of EPS and hyperprolactinemia, secondary to D2 receptor antagonism in the nigrostriatal and tuberoinfundibular pathways, respectively[1-3]. However, all SGAs also demonstrate affinity for serotonin 5-HT2a receptors, and antagonism at this site may subsequently increase release of dopamine and norepinephrine in the nigrostriatal and tuberoinfundibular pathways. This mechanism tends to counter the risk of these adverse events[3]. In addition, it is believed that antagonism of 5-HT2a receptors in the mesocortical pathway serves to ameliorate the negative symptoms of schizophrenia as well as mediate pro-cognitive benefits via increased dopaminergic activity[3,25,26].

Interestingly, some of the newer antipsychotics (aripiprazole, brexpiprazole, and cariprazine) have been found to mediate antipsychotic and antimanic efficacy through partial D2/D3 receptor *agonism*, and because of this unique mechanism are sometimes referred to as the third generation antipsychotics (TGA), or the *atypical* atypicals[208-211]. This partial agonism increases dopaminergic transmission in areas of *hypo*dopaminergic activity (mesocortical pathway) and dampens endogenous dopamine in areas of *hyper*dopaminergic activity (mesolimbic pathway), but not to the levels of a full agonist or antagonist, respectively. Theoretically, this partial dopamine agonism in the nigrostriatal and tuberoinfundibular pathways should be associated with a decreased risk of EPS and hyperprolactinemia. Aripiprazole and cariprazine however appear to carry a higher risk of akathisia[23,187,228], and all patients taking any SGA should therefore be educated and monitored for the development of EPS. It is possible, alternatively, that akathisia is mislabeled and these agitated, restless side effects may be due to increased serotonin activity, not unlike SSRI-induced agitation and activation.

More recently, some SGAs have demonstrated efficacy in the treatment of childhood schizophrenia and bipolar mania, autism, and depressive disorders (either as adjunct or monotherapy), and have been subsequently approved by the FDA for such use. Secondary to their complex and unique pharmacodynamic profiles, the SGAs are multifunctional drugs[246], and even without FDA approved indications, there appears to exist reasonable evidence (published randomized, placebo-controlled clinical trials, case reports, clinical experience) for their continued off-label use in depressive and anxiety disorders. Many of the non-dopaminergic properties that mediate such antidepressive and anxiolytic efficacy occur at much lower dosing ranges than needed for antipsychotic activity. As discussed in this review, some of these mechanisms (which differ with each antipsychotic) include serotonergic 5-HT1a partial agonism, and antagonism of the 5-HT2c, 5-HT6, 5-HT7, and α2-adrenergic receptors. In addition, at such low dosages, adverse events are less likely to occur, thereby allowing for safer treatment options and perhaps improved patient compliance.

In summary, the SGAs can be dosed flexibly as either monotherapies or as augmentation strategies based upon underlying patient symptoms and goals of treatment. At lower doses, these agents may be used as antidepressants/anxiolytics, while at higher doses they can be prescribed for their antipsychotic and antimanic efficacy. Although relatively safe if dosed judiciously and at appropriate levels, the SGAs always carry side effect risks, which varies and is largely dependent upon the unique pharmacodynamic profile of each agent. Patients should be routinely monitored for the development of not only EPS, TD, and cardiometabolic disorders, but for adverse events related to antagonism of histamine H1 receptors (sedation), muscarinic M1 receptors (constipation, urinary retention, blurry vision, and confusion/delirium), and α1-adrenergic receptors (dizziness and hypotension). As with any dosing strategy, clinicians should strive to achieve a careful balance between treatment efficacy and patient tolerability when prescribing the second and third generation antipsychotics.

REFERENCES

1   Kapur S, Zipursky R, Jones C, Remington G, Houle S. Relationship between dopamine D(2) occupancy, clinical response, and side effects: a double-blind PET study of first-episode schizophrenia. *The American journal of psychiatry.* 2000;157(4):514-20.

2   Glenthoj B, Mogensen J, Laursen H, Holm S, Hemmingsen R. Electrical sensitization of the meso-limbic dopaminergic system in rats: a pathogenetic model for schizophrenia. *Brain research.* 1993;619(1-2):39-54.

3   Stahl S. *Stahl's Essential Psychopharmacology: Neuroscientific Basis & Practical Applications.* . 4th ed: Cambridge University Press; 2013.

4   Sadock BJ, Sadock VA, Ruiz PR. *Kaplan and Sadock's synopsis of psychiatry.* 11th ed: Wolters Kluwer; 2015.

5   Edlinger M, Baumgartner S, Eltanaihi-Furtmuller N, Hummer M, Fleischhacker WW. Switching between second-generation antipsychotics: why and how? *CNS drugs.* 2005;19(1):27-42.

6   Citrome L, Jaffe A, Levine J. Dosing of second-generation antipsychotic medication in a state hospital system. *Journal of clinical psychopharmacology.* 2005;25(4):388-91.

7   Schwartz TL, Stahl SM. Treatment strategies for dosing the second generation antipsychotics. *CNS neuroscience & therapeutics.* 2011;17(2):110-7.

8   Citrome L, Volavka J. Optimal dosing of atypical antipsychotics in adults: a review of the current evidence. *Harvard review of psychiatry.* 2002;10(5):280-91.

9   Citrome L, Jaffe A, Levine J. How dosing of ziprasidone in a state hospital system differs from product labeling. *The Journal of clinical psychiatry.* 2009;70(7):975-82.

10   Citrome L, Kantrowitz JT. Olanzapine dosing above the licensed range is more efficacious than lower doses: fact or fiction? *Expert Rev Neurother.* 2009;9(7):1045-58.

11 Citrome L, Jaffe A, Levine J. Datapoints: The ups and downs of dosing second-generation antipsychotics. *Psychiatric services.* 2007;58(1):11.

12 Citrome L, Jaffe A, Levine J, Lindenmayer JP. Dosing of quetiapine in schizophrenia: how clinical practice differs from registration studies. *The Journal of clinical psychiatry.* 2005;66(12):1512-6.

13 Ishibashi T, Horisawa T, Tokuda K, Ishiyama T, Ogasa M, Tagashira R, Matsumoto K, Nishikawa H, Ueda Y, Toma S, Oki H, Tanno N, Saji I, Ito A, Ohno Y, Nakamura M. Pharmacological profile of lurasidone, a novel antipsychotic agent with potent 5-hydroxytryptamine 7 (5-HT7) and 5-HT1A receptor activity. *J Pharmacol Exp Ther.* 2010;334(1):171-81.

14 Maeda K, Lerdrup L, Sugino H, Akazawa H, Amada N, McQuade RD, Stensbol TB, Bundgaard C, Arnt J, Kikuchi T. Brexpiprazole II: antipsychotic-like and procognitive effects of a novel serotonin-dopamine activity modulator. *J Pharmacol Exp Ther.* 2014;350(3):605-14.

15 Maeda K, Sugino H, Akazawa H, Amada N, Shimada J, Futamura T, Yamashita H, Ito N, McQuade RD, Mork A, Pehrson AL, Hentzer M, Nielsen V, Bundgaard C, Arnt J, Stensbol TB, Kikuchi T. Brexpiprazole I: in vitro and in vivo characterization of a novel serotonin-dopamine activity modulator. *J Pharmacol Exp Ther.* 2014;350(3):589-604.

16 Kiss B, Horvath A, Nemethy Z, Schmidt E, Laszlovszky I, Bugovics G, Fazekas K, Hornok K, Orosz S, Gyertyan I, Agai-Csongor E, Domany G, Tihanyi K, Adham N, Szombathelyi Z. Cariprazine (RGH-188), a dopamine D(3) receptor-preferring, D(3)/D(2) dopamine receptor antagonist-partial agonist antipsychotic candidate: in vitro and neurochemical profile. *J Pharmacol Exp Ther.* 2010;333(1):328-40.

17 Roman V, Gyertyan I, Saghy K, Kiss B, Szombathelyi Z. Cariprazine (RGH-188), a D(3)-preferring dopamine D(3)/D(2) receptor partial agonist antipsychotic candidate demonstrates anti-abuse potential in rats. *Psychopharmacology.* 2013;226(2):285-93.

18 Macaluso M, Kazanchi H, Preskorn SH. How the pharmacokinetics and receptor-binding profile of lurasidone affect the clinical utility and safety of the drug in the treatment of schizophrenia. *Expert Opin Drug Metab Toxicol.* 2015;11(8):1317-27.

19 Citrome L. Iloperidone, asenapine, and lurasidone: a brief overview of 3 new second-generation antipsychotics. *Postgraduate medicine.* 2011;123(2):153-62.

20 Citrome L. Iloperidone: chemistry, pharmacodynamics, pharmacokinetics and metabolism, clinical efficacy, safety and tolerability, regulatory affairs, and an opinion. *Expert Opin Drug Metab Toxicol.* 2010;6(12):1551-64.

21 Shahid M, Walker GB, Zorn SH, Wong EH. Asenapine: a novel psychopharmacologic agent with a unique human receptor signature. *Journal of psychopharmacology.* 2009;23(1):65-73.

22 Citrome L. Asenapine review, part I: chemistry, receptor affinity profile, pharmacokinetics and metabolism. *Expert Opin Drug Metab Toxicol.* 2014;10(6):893-903.

23 Citrome L. The ABC's of dopamine receptor partial agonists - aripiprazole, brexpiprazole and cariprazine: the 15-min challenge to sort these agents out. *International journal of clinical practice.* 2015;69(11):1211-20.

24 Shayegan DK, Stahl SM. Atypical antipsychotics: matching receptor profile to individual patient's clinical profile. *CNS spectrums.* 2004;9(10 Suppl 11):6-14.

25 Schmidt CJ, Sorensen SM, Kehne JH, Carr AA, Palfreyman MG. The role of 5-HT2A receptors in antipsychotic activity. *Life Sci.* 1995;56(25):2209-22.

26 Akhondzadeh S, Malek-Hosseini M, Ghoreishi A, Raznahan M, Rezazadeh SA. Effect of ritanserin, a 5HT2A/2C antagonist, on negative symptoms of schizophrenia: a double-blind randomized placebo-controlled study. *Prog Neuropsychopharmacol Biol Psychiatry.* 2008;32(8):1879-83.

27 Sesack SR, Carr DB. Selective prefrontal cortex inputs to dopamine cells: implications for schizophrenia. *Physiol Behav.* 2002;77(4-5):513-7.

28 Blair DT, Dauner A. Extrapyramidal symptoms are serious side-effects of antipsychotic and other drugs. *Nurse Pract.* 1992;17(11):56, 62-4, 7.

29 Weiden PJ. EPS profiles: the atypical antipsychotics are not all the same. *Journal of psychiatric practice.* 2007;13(1):13-24.

30 Farah A. Atypicality of atypical antipsychotics. *Prim Care Companion J Clin Psychiatry.* 2005;7(6):268-74.

31 Compton MT, Miller AH. Antipsychotic-induced hyperprolactinemia and sexual dysfunction. *Psychopharmacol Bull.* 2002;36(1):143-64.

32 Meltzer HY, Matsubara S, Lee JC. Classification of typical and atypical antipsychotic drugs on the basis of dopamine D-1, D-2 and serotonin2 pKi values. *J Pharmacol Exp Ther.* 1989;251(1):238-46.

33 Kapur S, Seeman P. Does fast dissociation from the dopamine d(2) receptor explain the action of atypical antipsychotics?: A new hypothesis. *The American journal of psychiatry.* 2001;158(3):360-9.

34 Kapur S, Zipursky R, Jones C, Shammi CS, Remington G, Seeman P. A positron emission tomography study of quetiapine in schizophrenia: a preliminary finding of an antipsychotic effect with only transiently high dopamine D2 receptor occupancy. *Archives of general psychiatry.* 2000;57(6):553-9.

35 Stahl SM. "Hit-and-Run" actions at dopamine receptors, part 2: Illustrating fast dissociation from dopamine receptors that typifies atypical antipsychotics. *The Journal of clinical psychiatry.* 2001;62(10):747-8.

36 Bobes J, Rejas J, Garcia-Garcia M, Rico-Villademoros F, Garcia-Portilla MP, Fernandez I, Hernandez G, Group ES. Weight gain in patients with schizophrenia treated with risperidone, olanzapine, quetiapine or haloperidol: results of the EIRE study. *Schizophrenia research.* 2003;62(1-2):77-88.

37 Brooks JO, 3rd, Chang HS, Krasnykh O. Metabolic risks in older adults receiving second-generation antipsychotic medication. *Curr Psychiatry Rep.* 2009;11(1):33-40.

38 Leslie DL, Rosenheck RA. Incidence of newly diagnosed diabetes attributable to atypical antipsychotic medications. *The American journal of psychiatry.* 2004;161(9):1709-11.

39 Roerig JL, Steffen KJ, Mitchell JE. Atypical antipsychotic-induced weight gain: insights into mechanisms of action. *CNS drugs.* 2011;25(12):1035-59.

40 He M, Deng C, Huang XF. The role of hypothalamic H1 receptor antagonism in antipsychotic-induced weight gain. *CNS drugs.* 2013;27(6):423-34.

41 Provensi G, Blandina P, Passani MB. The histaminergic system as a target for the prevention of obesity and metabolic syndrome. *Neuropharmacology.* 2015;10.1016/j.neuropharm.2015.07.002.

42 Deng C, Weston-Green K, Huang XF. The role of histaminergic H1 and H3 receptors in food intake: a mechanism for atypical antipsychotic-induced weight gain? *Prog Neuropsychopharmacol Biol Psychiatry.* 2010;34(1):1-4.

43 Davoodi N, Kalinichev M, Clifton PG. Comparative effects of olanzapine and ziprasidone on hypophagia induced by enhanced histamine neurotransmission in the rat. *Behav Pharmacol.* 2008;19(2):121-8.

44 Stahl SM, Mignon L, Meyer JM. Which comes first: atypical antipsychotic treatment or cardiometabolic risk? *Acta Psychiatr Scand.* 2009;119(3):171-9.

45 Kroeze WK, Hufeisen SJ, Popadak BA, Renock SM, Steinberg S, Ernsberger P, Jayathilake K, Meltzer HY, Roth BL. H1-histamine receptor affinity predicts short-term weight gain for typical and atypical antipsychotic drugs. *Neuropsychopharmacology : official publication of the American College of Neuropsychopharmacology.* 2003;28(3):519-26.

46 Nonogaki K, Abdallah L, Goulding EH, Bonasera SJ, Tecott LH. Hyperactivity and reduced energy cost of physical activity in serotonin 5-HT(2C) receptor mutant mice. *Diabetes.* 2003;52(2):315-20.

47 Bickerdike MJ. 5-HT2C receptor agonists as potential drugs for the treatment of obesity. *Curr Top Med Chem.* 2003;3(8):885-97.

48 Kirk SL, Glazebrook J, Grayson B, Neill JC, Reynolds GP. Olanzapine-induced weight gain in the rat: role of 5-HT2C and histamine H1 receptors. *Psychopharmacology.* 2009;207(1):119-25.

49 Giorgetti M, Tecott LH. Contributions of 5-HT(2C) receptors to multiple actions of central serotonin systems. *Eur J Pharmacol.* 2004;488(1-3):1-9.

50 RISPERDAL (risperidone) tablet, RISPERDAL M-TAB (risperidone) tablet, orally disintegrating, RISPERDAL (risperidone) solution. Janssen Pharmaceuticals, Inc. DailyMed. Bethesda (MD): National Library

of Medicine (US). http://dailymed.nlm.nih.gov/dailymed/drugInfo. cfm?id=5420.

51   Haas M, Unis AS, Armenteros J, Copenhaver MD, Quiroz JA, Kushner SF. A 6-week, randomized, double-blind, placebo-controlled study of the efficacy and safety of risperidone in adolescents with schizophrenia. *J Child Adolesc Psychopharmacol.* 2009;19(6):611-21.

52   Pandina G, Kushner S, Karcher K, Haas M. An open-label, multicenter evaluation of the long-term safety and efficacy of risperidone in adolescents with schizophrenia. *Child Adolesc Psychiatry Ment Health.* 2012;6(1):23.

53   Khanna S, Vieta E, Lyons B, Grossman F, Eerdekens M, Kramer M. Risperidone in the treatment of acute mania: double-blind, placebo-controlled study. *The British journal of psychiatry : the journal of mental science.* 2005;187:229-34.

54   Scott LJ, Dhillon S. Risperidone: a review of its use in the treatment of irritability associated with autistic disorder in children and adolescents. *Paediatr Drugs.* 2007;9(5):343-54.

55   Han C, Wang SM, Kato M, Lee SJ, Patkar AA, Masand PS, Pae CU. Second-generation antipsychotics in the treatment of major depressive disorder: current evidence. *Expert Rev Neurother.* 2013;13(7):851-70.

56   Viner MW, Chen Y, Bakshi I, Kamper P. Low-dose risperidone augmentation of antidepressants in nonpsychotic depressive disorders with suicidal ideation. *Journal of clinical psychopharmacology.* 2003;23(1):104-6.

57   Ostroff RB, Nelson JC. Risperidone augmentation of selective serotonin reuptake inhibitors in major depression. *The Journal of clinical psychiatry.* 1999;60(4):256-9.

58   Rapaport MH, Gharabawi GM, Canuso CM, Mahmoud RA, Keller MB, Bossie CA, Turkoz I, Lasser RA, Loescher A, Bouhours P, Dunbar F, Nemeroff CB. Effects of risperidone augmentation in patients with treatment-resistant depression: Results of open-label treatment followed by double-blind continuation. *Neuropsychopharmacology : official publication of the American College of Neuropsychopharmacology.* 2006;31(11):2505-13.

59 Alexopoulos GS, Canuso CM, Gharabawi GM, Bossie CA, Greenspan A, Turkoz I, Reynolds C, 3rd. Placebo-controlled study of relapse prevention with risperidone augmentation in older patients with resistant depression. *Am J Geriatr Psychiatry.* 2008;16(1):21-30.

60 Mahmoud RA, Pandina GJ, Turkoz I, Kosik-Gonzalez C, Canuso CM, Kujawa MJ, Gharabawi-Garibaldi GM. Risperidone for treatment-refractory major depressive disorder: a randomized trial. *Ann Intern Med.* 2007;147(9):593-602.

61 Reeves H, Batra S, May RS, Zhang R, Dahl DC, Li X. Efficacy of risperidone augmentation to antidepressants in the management of suicidality in major depressive disorder: a randomized, double-blind, placebo-controlled pilot study. *The Journal of clinical psychiatry.* 2008;69(8):1228-336.

62 Keitner GI, Garlow SJ, Ryan CE, Ninan PT, Solomon DA, Nemeroff CB, Keller MB. A randomized, placebo-controlled trial of risperidone augmentation for patients with difficult-to-treat unipolar, non-psychotic major depression. *Journal of psychiatric research.* 2009;43(3):205-14.

63 Gabriel A. Risperidone, quetiapine, and olanzapine adjunctive treatments in major depression with psychotic features: a comparative study. *Neuropsychiatr Dis Treat.* 2013;9:485-92.

64 Yoshimura R, Umene-Nakano W, Ueda N, Ikenouchi-Sugita A, Hori H, Nakamura J. Addition of risperidone to sertraline improves sertraline-resistant refractory depression without influencing plasma concentrations of sertraline and desmethylsertraline. *Hum Psychopharmacol.* 2008;23(8):707-13.

65 Huang EJ, Reichardt LF. Neurotrophins: roles in neuronal development and function. *Annual review of neuroscience.* 2001;24:677-736.

66 Sen S, Duman R, Sanacora G. Serum brain-derived neurotrophic factor, depression, and antidepressant medications: meta-analyses and implications. *Biological psychiatry.* 2008;64(6):527-32.

67 Ray MT, Shannon Weickert C, Webster MJ. Decreased BDNF and TrkB mRNA expression in multiple cortical areas of patients with schizophrenia and mood disorders. *Transl Psychiatry.* 2014;4:e389.

68 Lee AH, Lange C, Ricken R, Hellweg R, Lang UE. Reduced brain-derived neurotrophic factor serum concentrations in acute schizophrenic patients increase during antipsychotic treatment. *Journal of clinical psychopharmacology.* 2011;31(3):334-6.

69 Angelucci F, Brene S, Mathe AA. BDNF in schizophrenia, depression and corresponding animal models. *Molecular psychiatry.* 2005;10(4):345-52.

70 Martinowich K, Lu B. Interaction between BDNF and serotonin: role in mood disorders. *Neuropsychopharmacology : official publication of the American College of Neuropsychopharmacology.* 2008;33(1):73-83.

71 Castren E, Rantamaki T. The role of BDNF and its receptors in depression and antidepressant drug action: Reactivation of developmental plasticity. *Developmental neurobiology.* 2010;70(5):289-97.

72 Brawman-Mintzer O, Knapp RG, Nietert PJ. Adjunctive risperidone in generalized anxiety disorder: a double-blind, placebo-controlled study. *The Journal of clinical psychiatry.* 2005;66(10):1321-5.

73 Simon NM, Hoge EA, Fischmann D, Worthington JJ, Christian KM, Kinrys G, Pollack MH. An open-label trial of risperidone augmentation for refractory anxiety disorders. *The Journal of clinical psychiatry.* 2006;67(3):381-5.

74 Pandina GJ, Canuso CM, Turkoz I, Kujawa M, Mahmoud RA. Adjunctive risperidone in the treatment of generalized anxiety disorder: a double-blind, prospective, placebo-controlled, randomized trial. *Psychopharmacol Bull.* 2007;40(3):41-57.

75 Sheehan DV, McElroy SL, Harnett-Sheehan K, Keck PE, Jr., Janavs J, Rogers J, Gonzalez R, Shivakumar G, Suppes T. Randomized, placebo-controlled trial of risperidone for acute treatment of bipolar anxiety. *J Affect Disord.* 2009;115(3):376-85.

76 Pira L, Mongeau R, Pani L. The atypical antipsychotic quetiapine increases both noradrenaline and dopamine release in the rat prefrontal cortex. *Eur J Pharmacol.* 2004;504(1-2):61-4.

77 Blier P, Szabo ST. Potential mechanisms of action of atypical antipsychotic medications in treatment-resistant depression and anxiety. *The Journal of clinical psychiatry.* 2005;66 Suppl 8:30-40.

78 Hedlund PB. The 5-HT7 receptor and disorders of the nervous system: an overview. *Psychopharmacology.* 2009;206(3):345-54.

79 Waters KA, Stean TO, Hammond B, Virley DJ, Upton N, Kew JN, Hussain I. Effects of the selective 5-HT(7) receptor antagonist SB-269970 in animal models of psychosis and cognition. *Behav Brain Res.* 2012;228(1):211-8.

80 Saito E, Correll CU, Gallelli K, McMeniman M, Parikh UH, Malhotra AK, Kafantaris V. A prospective study of hyperprolactinemia in children and adolescents treated with atypical antipsychotic agents. *J Child Adolesc Psychopharmacol.* 2004;14(3):350-8.

81 Kapur S, Langlois X, Vinken P, Megens AA, De Coster R, Andrews JS. The differential effects of atypical antipsychotics on prolactin elevation are explained by their differential blood-brain disposition: a pharmacological analysis in rats. *J Pharmacol Exp Ther.* 2002;302(3):1129-34.

82 Kapur S, Roy P, Daskalakis J, Remington G, Zipursky R. Increased dopamine d(2) receptor occupancy and elevated prolactin level associated with addition of haloperidol to clozapine. *The American journal of psychiatry.* 2001;158(2):311-4.

83 Knegtering R, Baselmans P, Castelein S, Bosker F, Bruggeman R, van den Bosch RJ. Predominant role of the 9-hydroxy metabolite of risperidone in elevating blood prolactin levels. *The American journal of psychiatry.* 2005;162(5):1010-2.

84 INVEGA (paliperidone) tablet, extended release. DailyMed. Bethesda (MD): National Library of Medicine (US). http://dailymed.nlm.nih.gov/dailymed/drugInfo.cfm?id=5420.

85 Yang FW, Liang CS. Paliperidone augmentation for treatment-resistant depression: a case report. *Journal of clinical psychopharmacology.* 2011;31(2):245-6.

86 Turkoz I, Bossie CA, Lindenmayer JP, Schooler N, Canuso CM. Paliperidone ER and oral risperidone in patients with schizophrenia: a comparative database analysis. *BMC Psychiatry.* 2011;11:21.

87 Hou YC, Lai CH. Lower risk for body weight gain and better control of appetite after switching risperidone to paliperidone in a schizoaffective patient. *J Neuropsychiatry Clin Neurosci.* 2014;26(2):E36-7.

88   GEODON- ziprasidone hydrochloride capsule GEODON- ziprasidone
     mesylate injection, powder, lyophilized, for solution DailyMed. Bethesda
     (MD): National Library of Medicine (US). http://dailymed.nlm.nih.gov/
     dailymed/drugInfo.cfm?id=5420.

89   Keck PE, Jr., McElroy SL, Arnold LM. Ziprasidone: a new atypical
     antipsychotic. *Expert Opin Pharmacother.* 2001;2(6):1033-42.

90   Warrington L, Lombardo I, Loebel A, Ice K. Ziprasidone for the treatment
     of acute manic or mixed episodes associated with bipolar disorder. *CNS
     drugs.* 2007;21(10):835-49.

91   Addington DE, Labelle A, Kulkarni J, Johnson G, Loebel A, Mandel FS.
     A comparison of ziprasidone and risperidone in the long-term treatment
     of schizophrenia: a 44-week, double-blind, continuation study. *Can J
     Psychiatry.* 2009;54(1):46-54.

92   Sciarretta A, Piazzi G. Long-term safety of ziprasidone in schizophrenic
     patients: an open trial. *Eur Rev Med Pharmacol Sci.* 2012;16(15):2113-9.

93   Findling RL, Cavus I, Pappadopulos E, Vanderburg DG, Schwartz
     JH, Gundapaneni BK, DelBello MP. Ziprasidone in adolescents
     with schizophrenia: results from a placebo-controlled efficacy and
     long-term open-extension study. *J Child Adolesc Psychopharmacol.*
     2013;23(8):531-44.

94   Findling RL, Cavus I, Pappadopulos E, Vanderburg DG, Schwartz JH,
     Gundapaneni BK, DelBello MP. Efficacy, long-term safety, and tolerability
     of ziprasidone in children and adolescents with bipolar disorder. *J Child
     Adolesc Psychopharmacol.* 2013;23(8):545-57.

95   Citrome L, Reist C, Palmer L, Montejano LB, Lenhart G, Cuffel B, Harnett
     J, Sanders KN. Impact of real-world ziprasidone dosing on treatment
     discontinuation rates in patients with schizophrenia or bipolar disorder.
     Schizophrenia research. 2009;115(2-3):115-20.

96   Stahl S, Lombardo I, Loebel A, Mandel FS. Efficacy of ziprasidone in
     dysphoric mania: pooled analysis of two double-blind studies. *J Affect
     Disord.* 2010;122(1-2):39-45.

97   Cutler A, Ball S, Stahl SM. Dosing atypical antipsychotics. *CNS
     spectrums.* 2008;13(5 Suppl 9):1-16.

98 Papakostas GI, Vitolo OV, Ishak WW, Rapaport MH, Zajecka JM, Kinrys G, Mischoulon D, Lipkin SH, Hails KA, Abrams J, Ward SG, Meisner A, Schoenfeld DA, Shelton RC, Winokur A, Okasha MS, Bari MA, Fava M. A 12-week, randomized, double-blind, placebo-controlled, sequential parallel comparison trial of ziprasidone as monotherapy for major depressive disorder. *The Journal of clinical psychiatry.* 2012;73(12):1541-7.

99 Sachs GS, Ice KS, Chappell PB, Schwartz JH, Gurtovaya O, Vanderburg DG, Kasuba B. Efficacy and safety of adjunctive oral ziprasidone for acute treatment of depression in patients with bipolar I disorder: a randomized, double-blind, placebo-controlled trial. *The Journal of clinical psychiatry.* 2011;72(10):1413-22.

100 Liebowitz MR, Salman E, Mech A, Dunner D, Johnson AE, Akhtar J, Pratap R. Ziprasidone monotherapy in bipolar II depression: an open trial. *J Affect Disord.* 2009;118(1-3):205-8.

101 Rosa AR, Franco C, Torrent C, Comes M, Cruz N, Horga G, Benabarre A, Vieta E. Ziprasidone in the treatment of affective disorders: a review. *CNS neuroscience & therapeutics.* 2008;14(4):278-86.

102 Snyderman SH, Rynn MA, Rickels K. Open-label pilot study of ziprasidone for refractory generalized anxiety disorder. *Journal of clinical psychopharmacology.* 2005;25(5):497-9.

103 Papakostas GI, Petersen TJ, Nierenberg AA, Murakami JL, Alpert JE, Rosenbaum JF, Fava M. Ziprasidone augmentation of selective serotonin reuptake inhibitors (SSRIs) for SSRI-resistant major depressive disorder. *The Journal of clinical psychiatry.* 2004;65(2):217-21.

104 Dunner DL, Amsterdam JD, Shelton RC, Loebel A, Romano SJ. Efficacy and tolerability of adjunctive ziprasidone in treatment-resistant depression: a randomized, open-label, pilot study. *The Journal of clinical psychiatry.* 2007;68(7):1071-7.

105 Papakostas GI, Fava M, Baer L, Swee MB, Jaeger A, Bobo WV, Shelton RC. Ziprasidone Augmentation of Escitalopram for Major Depressive Disorder: Efficacy Results From a Randomized, Double-Blind, Placebo-Controlled Study. *The American journal of psychiatry.* 2015;172(12):1251-8.

106 Stahl SM, Shayegan DK. The psychopharmacology of ziprasidone: receptor-binding properties and real-world psychiatric practice. *The Journal of clinical psychiatry.* 2003;64 Suppl 19:6-12.

107 Dremencov E, Newman ME, Kinor N, Blatman-Jan G, Schindler CJ, Overstreet DH, Yadid G. Hyperfunctionality of serotonin-2C receptor-mediated inhibition of accumbal dopamine release in an animal model of depression is reversed by antidepressant treatment. *Neuropharmacology.* 2005;48(1):34-42.

108 Jahanshahi A, Lim LW, Steinbusch HW, Visser-Vandewalle V, Temel Y. Buspirone-induced changes in the serotonergic and non-serotonergic cells in the dorsal raphe nucleus of rats. *Neuroscience letters.* 2010;473(2):136-40.

109 De Vry J, Schreiber R, Melon C, Dalmus M, Jentzsch KR. 5-HT1A receptors are differentially involved in the anxiolytic- and antidepressant-like effects of 8-OH-DPAT and fluoxetine in the rat. *European neuropsychopharmacology : the journal of the European College of Neuropsychopharmacology.* 2004;14(6):487-95.

110 Edwards SJ, Smith CJ. Tolerability of atypical antipsychotics in the treatment of adults with schizophrenia or bipolar disorder: a mixed treatment comparison of randomized controlled trials. *Clin Ther.* 2009;31 Pt 1:1345-59.

111 Camm AJ, Karayal ON, Meltzer H, Kolluri S, O'Gorman C, Miceli J, Tensfeldt T, Kane JM. Ziprasidone and the corrected QT interval: a comprehensive summary of clinical data. *CNS drugs.* 2012;26(4):351-65.

112 FANAPT (iloperidone) tablet, FANAPT (iloperidone) kit DailyMed. Bethesda (MD): National Library of Medicine (US). http://dailymed.nlm.nih.gov/dailymed/drugInfo.cfm?id=5420.

113 Scott LJ. Iloperidone: in schizophrenia. *CNS drugs.* 2009;23(10):867-80.

114 Cutler AJ. Iloperidone: a new option for the treatment of schizophrenia. *Expert Rev Neurother.* 2009;9(12):1727-41.

115 Kane JM, Lauriello J, Laska E, Di Marino M, Wolfgang CD. Long-term efficacy and safety of iloperidone: results from 3 clinical trials for the treatment of schizophrenia. *Journal of clinical psychopharmacology.* 2008;28(2 Suppl 1):S29-35.

116 Subramanian N, Kalkman HO. Receptor profile of P88-8991 and P95-12113, metabolites of the novel antipsychotic iloperidone. *Prog Neuropsychopharmacol Biol Psychiatry.* 2002;26(3):553-60.

117 Ionescu DF, Fava M, Ju Hyung Kim D, Baer L, Shelton RC, Cusin C. A placebo-controlled crossover study of iloperidone augmentation for residual anger and irritability in major depressive disorder. *Therapeutic Advances in Psychopharmacology.* 2015;10.1177/2045125315618621.

118 Iloperidone in Mixed States of Bipolar Disorder. ClinicalTrials.gov [Internet]. Bethesda (MD): National Library of Medicine (US). 2015-[cited 2016 Jan 22]. https://clinicaltrials.gov/ct2/show/NCT02413918.

119 Citrome L. Iloperidone redux: a dissection of the Drug Approval Package for this newly commercialised second-generation antipsychotic. *International journal of clinical practice.* 2010;64(6):707-18.

120 Wesolowska A. Potential role of the 5-HT6 receptor in depression and anxiety: an overview of preclinical data. *Pharmacol Rep.* 2010;62(4):564-77.

121 Potkin SG, Preskorn S, Hochfeld M, Meng X. A thorough QTc study of 3 doses of iloperidone including metabolic inhibition via CYP2D6 and/or CYP3A4 and a comparison to quetiapine and ziprasidone. *Journal of clinical psychopharmacology.* 2013;33(1):3-10.

122 LATUDA- lurasidone hydrochloride tablet, film coated DailyMed. Bethesda (MD): National Library of Medicine (US). http://dailymed.nlm.nih.gov/dailymed/drugInfo.cfm?id=5420.

123 Loebel A, Cucchiaro J, Xu J, Sarma K, Pikalov A, Kane JM. Effectiveness of lurasidone vs. quetiapine XR for relapse prevention in schizophrenia: a 12-month, double-blind, noninferiority study. *Schizophrenia research.* 2013;147(1):95-102.

124 Citrome L, Cucchiaro J, Sarma K, Phillips D, Silva R, Tsuchiya S, Loebel A. Long-term safety and tolerability of lurasidone in schizophrenia: a 12-month, double-blind, active-controlled study. *International clinical psychopharmacology.* 2012;27(3):165-76.

125 Preskorn S, Ereshefsky L, Chiu YY, Poola N, Loebel A. Effect of food on the pharmacokinetics of lurasidone: results of two randomized, open-label, crossover studies. *Hum Psychopharmacol.* 2013;28(5):495-505.

126 Loebel A, Cucchiaro J, Silva R, Kroger H, Hsu J, Sarma K, Sachs G. Lurasidone monotherapy in the treatment of bipolar I depression: a randomized, double-blind, placebo-controlled study. *The American journal of psychiatry.* 2014;171(2):160-8.

127 Nasrallah HA, Cucchiaro JB, Mao Y, Pikalov AA, Loebel AD. Lurasidone for the treatment of depressive symptoms in schizophrenia: analysis of 4 pooled, 6-week, placebo-controlled studies. *CNS spectrums.* 2015;20(2):140-7.

128 A Randomized, 6-Week, Double-Blind, Placebo-Controlled, Flexible-Dose, Parallel-Group Study of Lurasidone for the Treatment of Major Depressive Disorder With Mixed Features. ClinicalTrials.gov [Internet]. Bethesda (MD): National Library of Medicine (US). 2015-[cited 2016 Jan 22]. https://clinicaltrials.gov/ct2/show/NCT01421134.

129 A 12-Week, Open-Label Extension Study For the Treatment of Major Depressive Disorder With Mixed Features. ClinicalTrials.gov [Internet]. Bethesda (MD): National Library of Medicine (US). 2015-[cited 2016 Jan 22]. https://clinicaltrials.gov/ct2/show/NCT01423253.

130 PL Detail-Document #281006: Comparison of Atypical Antipsychotics. In: Center TR, ed2012.

131 McDonagh M, Peterson K, Carson S, Fu R, Thakurta S. *Drug Class Review: Atypical Antipsychotic Drugs: Final Update 3 Report.* Portland (OR)2010.

132 Loebel A, Citrome L. Lurasidone: a novel antipsychotic agent for the treatment of schizophrenia and bipolar depression. *BJPsych Bull.* 2015;39(5):237-41.

133 Potkin SG, Ogasa M, Cucchiaro J, Loebel A. Double-blind comparison of the safety and efficacy of lurasidone and ziprasidone in clinically stable outpatients with schizophrenia or schizoaffective disorder. *Schizophrenia research.* 2011;132(2-3):101-7.

134 Rummel-Kluge C, Komossa K, Schwarz S, Hunger H, Schmid F, Lobos CA, Kissling W, Davis JM, Leucht S. Head-to-head comparisons of metabolic side effects of second generation antipsychotics in the treatment of schizophrenia: a systematic review and meta-analysis. *Schizophrenia research.* 2010;123(2-3):225-33.

135 Werner FM, Covenas R. Safety of antipsychotic drugs: focus on therapeutic and adverse effects. *Expert Opin Drug Saf.* 2014;13(8):1031-42.

136 Citrome L. Lurasidone for schizophrenia: a review of the efficacy and safety profile for this newly approved second-generation antipsychotic. *International journal of clinical practice.* 2011;65(2):189-210.

137 Stahl SM, Cucchiaro J, Simonelli D, Hsu J, Pikalov A, Loebel A. Effectiveness of lurasidone for patients with schizophrenia following 6 weeks of acute treatment with lurasidone, olanzapine, or placebo: a 6-month, open-label, extension study. *The Journal of clinical psychiatry.* 2013;74(5):507-15.

138 Chen Y, Bobo WV, Watts K, Jayathilake K, Tang T, Meltzer HY. Comparative effectiveness of switching antipsychotic drug treatment to aripiprazole or ziprasidone for improving metabolic profile and atherogenic dyslipidemia: a 12-month, prospective, open-label study. *Journal of psychopharmacology.* 2012;26(9):1201-10.

139 Park S, Yi KK, Kim MS, Hong JP. Effects of ziprasidone and olanzapine on body composition and metabolic parameters: an open-label comparative pilot study. *Behav Brain Funct.* 2013;9:27.

140 ZYPREXA - olanzapine tablet ZYPREXA ZYDIS - olanzapine tablet, orally disintegrating ZYPREXA INTRAMUSCULAR - olanzapine injection, powder, for solution. DailyMed. Bethesda (MD): National Library of Medicine (US). http://dailymed.nlm.nih.gov/dailymed/drugInfo. cfm?id=5420.

141 Burton ME, Shaw LM, Schentag JJ, Evans WE. *Applied Pharmacokinetics & Pharmacodynamics: Principles of Therapeutic Drug Monitoring.* 4th ed: Lippincott Williams & Williams; May 1, 2005.

142 Citrome L, Stauffer VL, Chen L, Kinon BJ, Kurtz DL, Jacobson JG, Bergstrom RF. Olanzapine plasma concentrations after treatment with 10, 20, and 40 mg/d in patients with schizophrenia: an analysis of correlations

with efficacy, weight gain, and prolactin concentration. *Journal of clinical psychopharmacology.* 2009;29(3):278-83.

143 Kinon BJ, Volavka J, Stauffer V, Edwards SE, Liu-Seifert H, Chen L, Adams DH, Lindenmayer JP, McEvoy JP, Buckley PF, Lieberman JA, Meltzer HY, Wilson DR, Citrome L. Standard and higher dose of olanzapine in patients with schizophrenia or schizoaffective disorder: a randomized, double-blind, fixed-dose study. *Journal of clinical psychopharmacology.* 2008;28(4):392-400.

144 Bobo WV, Epstein RA, Shelton RC. Olanzapine monotherapy for acute depression in patients with bipolar I or II disorder: results of an 8-week open label trial. *Hum Psychopharmacol.* 2010;25(1):30-6.

145 Corya SA, Perlis RH, Keck PE, Jr., Lin DY, Case MG, Williamson DJ, Tohen MF. A 24-week open-label extension study of olanzapine-fluoxetine combination and olanzapine monotherapy in the treatment of bipolar depression. *The Journal of clinical psychiatry.* 2006;67(5):798-806.

146 Tohen M, Kanba S, McIntyre RS, Fujikoshi S, Katagiri H. Efficacy of olanzapine monotherapy in the treatment of bipolar depression with mixed features. *J Affect Disord.* 2014;164:57-62.

147 Tohen M, Katagiri H, Fujikoshi S, Kanba S. Efficacy of olanzapine monotherapy in acute bipolar depression: a pooled analysis of controlled studies. *J Affect Disord.* 2013;149(1-3):196-201.

148 Wang M, Tong JH, Huang DS, Zhu G, Liang GM, Du H. Efficacy of olanzapine monotherapy for treatment of bipolar I depression: a randomized, double-blind, placebo controlled study. *Psychopharmacology.* 2014;231(14):2811-8.

149 Mathews J, Garcia KS, Mintun MA, Sheline YI. Antidepressant efficacy of olanzapine as monotherapy in major depressive disorder, without psychosis: a pilot study. *Psychiatry research.* 2006;146(2):149-55.

150 Shelton RC, Tollefson GD, Tohen M, Stahl S, Gannon KS, Jacobs TG, Buras WR, Bymaster FP, Zhang W, Spencer KA, Feldman PD, Meltzer HY. A novel augmentation strategy for treating resistant major depression. *The American journal of psychiatry.* 2001;158(1):131-4.

151 Shelton RC, Williamson DJ, Corya SA, Sanger TM, Van Campen LE, Case M, Briggs SD, Tollefson GD. Olanzapine/fluoxetine combination for treatment-resistant depression: a controlled study of SSRI and nortriptyline resistance. *The Journal of clinical psychiatry.* 2005;66(10):1289-97.

152 Corya SA, Williamson D, Sanger TM, Briggs SD, Case M, Tollefson G. A randomized, double-blind comparison of olanzapine/fluoxetine combination, olanzapine, fluoxetine, and venlafaxine in treatment-resistant depression. *Depress Anxiety.* 2006;23(6):364-72.

153 Meyers BS, Flint AJ, Rothschild AJ, Mulsant BH, Whyte EM, Peasley-Miklus C, Papademetriou E, Leon AC, Heo M, Group S-P. A double-blind randomized controlled trial of olanzapine plus sertraline vs olanzapine plus placebo for psychotic depression: the study of pharmacotherapy of psychotic depression (STOP-PD). *Archives of general psychiatry.* 2009;66(8):838-47.

154 Rothschild AJ, Williamson DJ, Tohen MF, Schatzberg A, Andersen SW, Van Campen LE, Sanger TM, Tollefson GD. A double-blind, randomized study of olanzapine and olanzapine/fluoxetine combination for major depression with psychotic features. *Journal of clinical psychopharmacology.* 2004;24(4):365-73.

155 Thase ME, Corya SA, Osuntokun O, Case M, Henley DB, Sanger TM, Watson SB, Dube S. A randomized, double-blind comparison of olanzapine/fluoxetine combination, olanzapine, and fluoxetine in treatment-resistant major depressive disorder. *The Journal of clinical psychiatry.* 2007;68(2):224-36.

156 Croxtall JD, Scott LJ. Olanzapine/fluoxetine: a review of its use in patients with treatment-resistant major depressive disorder. *CNS drugs.* 2010;24(3):245-62.

157 Barnett SD, Kramer ML, Casat CD, Connor KM, Davidson JR. Efficacy of olanzapine in social anxiety disorder: a pilot study. *Journal of psychopharmacology.* 2002;16(4):365-8.

158 Locchi F, Dall'olio R, Gandolfi O, Rimondini R. Olanzapine counteracts stress-induced anxiety-like behavior in rats. *Neuroscience letters.* 2008;438(2):146-9.

159 Pollack MH, Simon NM, Zalta AK, Worthington JJ, Hoge EA, Mick E, Kinrys G, Oppenheimer J. Olanzapine augmentation of fluoxetine for refractory generalized anxiety disorder: a placebo controlled study. *Biological psychiatry.* 2006;59(3):211-5.

160 McEvoy JP, Lieberman JA, Stroup TS, Davis SM, Meltzer HY, Rosenheck RA, Swartz MS, Perkins DO, Keefe RS, Davis CE, Severe J, Hsiao JK, Investigators C. Effectiveness of clozapine versus olanzapine, quetiapine, and risperidone in patients with chronic schizophrenia who did not respond to prior atypical antipsychotic treatment. *The American journal of psychiatry.* 2006;163(4):600-10.

161 SEROQUEL XR- quetiapine fumarate tablet, extended release SEROQUEL XR- quetiapine fumarate. DailyMed. Bethesda (MD): National Library of Medicine (US). http://dailymed.nlm.nih.gov/dailymed/drugInfo.cfm?id=5420.

162 Narala A, Veerabrahma K. Preparation, Characterization and Evaluation of Quetiapine Fumarate Solid Lipid Nanoparticles to Improve the Oral Bioavailability. *J Pharm (Cairo).* 2013;2013:265741.

163 Chaput Y, Magnan A, Gendron A. The co-administration of quetiapine or placebo to cognitive-behavior therapy in treatment refractory depression: a preliminary trial. *BMC Psychiatry.* 2008;8:73.

164 Bauer M, Pretorius HW, Constant EL, Earley WR, Szamosi J, Brecher M. Extended-release quetiapine as adjunct to an antidepressant in patients with major depressive disorder: results of a randomized, placebo-controlled, double-blind study. *The Journal of clinical psychiatry.* 2009;70(4):540-9.

165 El-Khalili N, Joyce M, Atkinson S, Buynak RJ, Datto C, Lindgren P, Eriksson H. Extended-release quetiapine fumarate (quetiapine XR) as adjunctive therapy in major depressive disorder (MDD) in patients with an inadequate response to ongoing antidepressant treatment: a multicentre, randomized, double-blind, placebo-controlled study. *The international journal of neuropsychopharmacology / official scientific journal of the Collegium Internationale Neuropsychopharmacologicum.* 2010;13(7):917-32.

166 McIntyre A, Gendron A, McIntyre A. Quetiapine adjunct to selective serotonin reuptake inhibitors or venlafaxine in patients with major depression, comorbid anxiety, and residual depressive symptoms: a randomized, placebo-controlled pilot study. *Depress Anxiety.* 2007;24(7):487-94.

167 Garakani A, Martinez JM, Marcus S, Weaver J, Rickels K, Fava M, Hirschowitz J. A randomized, double-blind, and placebo-controlled trial of quetiapine augmentation of fluoxetine in major depressive disorder. *International clinical psychopharmacology.* 2008;23(5):269-75.

168 Wijkstra J, Burger H, van den Broek WW, Birkenhager TK, Janzing JG, Boks MP, Bruijn JA, van der Loos ML, Breteler LM, Ramaekers GM, Verkes RJ, Nolen WA. Treatment of unipolar psychotic depression: a randomized, double-blind study comparing imipramine, venlafaxine, and venlafaxine plus quetiapine. *Acta Psychiatr Scand.* 2010;121(3):190-200.

169 Bortnick B, El-Khalili N, Banov M, Adson D, Datto C, Raines S, Earley W, Eriksson H. Efficacy and tolerability of extended release quetiapine fumarate (quetiapine XR) monotherapy in major depressive disorder: a placebo-controlled, randomized study. *J Affect Disord.* 2011;128(1-2):83-94.

170 Weisler R, Joyce M, McGill L, Lazarus A, Szamosi J, Eriksson H, Moonstone Study G. Extended release quetiapine fumarate monotherapy for major depressive disorder: results of a double-blind, randomized, placebo-controlled study. *CNS spectrums.* 2009;14(6):299-313.

171 Cutler AJ, Montgomery SA, Feifel D, Lazarus A, Astrom M, Brecher M. Extended release quetiapine fumarate monotherapy in major depressive disorder: a placebo- and duloxetine-controlled study. *The Journal of clinical psychiatry.* 2009;70(4):526-39.

172 Katila H, Mezhebovsky I, Mulroy A, Berggren L, Eriksson H, Earley W, Datto C. Randomized, double-blind study of the efficacy and tolerability of extended release quetiapine fumarate (quetiapine XR) monotherapy in elderly patients with major depressive disorder. *Am J Geriatr Psychiatry.* 2013;21(8):769-84.

173 Wang G, McIntyre A, Earley WR, Raines SR, Eriksson H. A randomized, double-blind study of the efficacy and tolerability of extended-release quetiapine fumarate (quetiapine XR) monotherapy in patients with major depressive disorder. *Neuropsychiatr Dis Treat.* 2014;10:201-16.

174 Kreys TJ, Phan SV. A literature review of quetiapine for generalized anxiety disorder. *Pharmacotherapy.* 2015;35(2):175-88.

175 Maneeton N, Maneeton B, Woottiluk P, Likhitsathian S, Suttajit S, Boonyanaruthee V, Srisurapanont M. Quetiapine monotherapy in acute treatment of generalized anxiety disorder: a systematic review and meta-analysis of randomized controlled trials. *Drug Des Devel Ther.* 2016;10:259-76.

176 SAPHRIS- asenapine maleate tablet DailyMed. Bethesda (MD): National Library of Medicine (US). http://dailymed.nlm.nih.gov/dailymed/drugInfo. cfm?id=5420.

177 Potkin SG, Phiri P, Szegedi A, Zhao J, Alphs L, Cazorla P. Long-term effects of asenapine or olanzapine in patients with persistent negative symptoms of schizophrenia: a pooled analysis. *Schizophrenia research.* 2013;150(2-3):442-9.

178 Schoemaker J, Naber D, Vrijland P, Panagides J, Emsley R. Long-term assessment of Asenapine vs. Olanzapine in patients with schizophrenia or schizoaffective disorder. *Pharmacopsychiatry.* 2010;43(4):138-46.

179 Schoemaker J, Stet L, Vrijland P, Naber D, Panagides J, Emsley R. Long-term efficacy and safety of asenapine or olanzapine in patients with schizophrenia or schizoaffective disorder: an extension study. *Pharmacopsychiatry.* 2012;45(5):196-203.

180 Kane JM, Mackle M, Snow-Adami L, Zhao J, Szegedi A, Panagides J. A randomized placebo-controlled trial of asenapine for the prevention of relapse of schizophrenia after long-term treatment. *The Journal of clinical psychiatry.* 2011;72(3):349-55.

181 McIntyre RS, Cohen M, Zhao J, Alphs L, Macek TA, Panagides J. Asenapine for long-term treatment of bipolar disorder: a double-blind 40-week extension study. *J Affect Disord.* 2010;126(3):358-65.

182 Asenapine for Bipolar Depression. ClinicalTrials.gov [Internet]. Bethesda (MD): National Library of Medicine (US). 2015-[cited 2016 Jan 22]. https:// clinicaltrials.gov/ct2/show/NCT01670019.

183 Antidepressant Plus Asenapine Versus Antidepressant Plus Placebo for Depression. ClinicalTrials.gov [Internet]. Bethesda (MD): National Library of Medicine (US). 2015-[cited 2016 Jan 22]. https://clinicaltrials.gov/ct2/ show/NCT01670019.

184 Ene HM, Kara NZ, Barak N, Reshef Ben-Mordechai T, Einat H. Effects of repeated asenapine in a battery of tests for anxiety-like behaviours in mice. *Acta Neuropsychiatr.* 2015;10.1017/neu.2015.53:1-7.

185 Citrome L. Asenapine review, part II: clinical efficacy, safety and tolerability. *Expert Opin Drug Saf.* 2014;13(6):803-30.

186 Franberg O, Marcus MM, Ivanov V, Schilstrom B, Shahid M, Svensson TH. Asenapine elevates cortical dopamine, noradrenaline and serotonin release. Evidence for activation of cortical and subcortical dopamine systems by different mechanisms. *Psychopharmacology.* 2009;204(2):251-64.

187 ABILIFY- aripiprazole tablet ABILIFY- aripiprazole solution ABILIFY- aripiprazole tablet, orally disintegrating ABILIFY- aripiprazole injection, solution. DailyMed. Bethesda (MD): National Library of Medicine (US). http://dailymed.nlm.nih.gov/dailymed/drugInfo.cfm?id=5420.

188 Papakostas GI, Petersen TJ, Kinrys G, Burns AM, Worthington JJ, Alpert JE, Fava M, Nierenberg AA. Aripiprazole augmentation of selective serotonin reuptake inhibitors for treatment-resistant major depressive disorder. *The Journal of clinical psychiatry.* 2005;66(10):1326-30.

189 Simon JS, Nemeroff CB. Aripiprazole augmentation of antidepressants for the treatment of partially responding and nonresponding patients with major depressive disorder. *The Journal of clinical psychiatry.* 2005;66(10):1216-20.

190 Patkar AA, Peindl K, Mago R, Mannelli P, Masand PS. An open-label, rater-blinded, augmentation study of aripiprazole in treatment-resistant depression. *Prim Care Companion J Clin Psychiatry.* 2006;8(2):82-7.

191 Rutherford B, Sneed J, Miyazaki M, Eisenstadt R, Devanand D, Sackeim H, Roose S. An open trial of aripiprazole augmentation for SSRI non-remitters with late-life depression. *Int J Geriatr Psychiatry.* 2007;22(10):986-91.

192 Worthington JJ, 3rd, Kinrys G, Wygant LE, Pollack MH. Aripiprazole as an augmentor of selective serotonin reuptake inhibitors in depression and anxiety disorder patients. *International clinical psychopharmacology.* 2005;20(1):9-11.

193 Hellerstein DJ, Batchelder S, Hyler S, Arnaout B, Corpuz V, Coram L, Weiss G. Aripiprazole as an adjunctive treatment for refractory unipolar depression. *Prog Neuropsychopharmacol Biol Psychiatry.* 2008;32(3):744-50.

194 Berman RM, Marcus RN, Swanink R, McQuade RD, Carson WH, Corey-Lisle PK, Khan A. The efficacy and safety of aripiprazole as adjunctive therapy in major depressive disorder: a multicenter, randomized, double-blind, placebo-controlled study. *The Journal of clinical psychiatry.* 2007;68(6):843-53.

195 Marcus RN, McQuade RD, Carson WH, Hennicken D, Fava M, Simon JS, Trivedi MH, Thase ME, Berman RM. The efficacy and safety of aripiprazole as adjunctive therapy in major depressive disorder: a second multicenter, randomized, double-blind, placebo-controlled study. *Journal of clinical psychopharmacology.* 2008;28(2):156-65.

196 Berman RM, Fava M, Thase ME, Trivedi MH, Swanink R, McQuade RD, Carson WH, Adson D, Taylor L, Hazel J, Marcus RN. Aripiprazole augmentation in major depressive disorder: a double-blind, placebo-controlled study in patients with inadequate response to antidepressants. *CNS spectrums.* 2009;14(4):197-206.

197 Fava M, Mischoulon D, Iosifescu D, Witte J, Pencina M, Flynn M, Harper L, Levy M, Rickels K, Pollack M. A double-blind, placebo-controlled study of aripiprazole adjunctive to antidepressant therapy among depressed outpatients with inadequate response to prior antidepressant therapy (ADAPT-A Study). *Psychother Psychosom.* 2012;81(2):87-97.

198 Mischoulon D, Witte J, Levy M, Papakostas GI, Pet LR, Hsieh WH, Pencina MJ, Ward S, Pollack MH, Fava M. Efficacy of dose increase among nonresponders to low-dose aripiprazole augmentation in patients with inadequate response to antidepressant treatment: a randomized, double-blind, placebo-controlled, efficacy trial. *The Journal of clinical psychiatry.* 2012;73(3):353-7.

199 Berman RM, Thase ME, Trivedi MH, Hazel JA, Marler SV, McQuade RD, Carson W, Baker RA, Marcus RN. Long-term safety and tolerability of open-label aripiprazole augmentation of antidepressant therapy in major depressive disorder. *Neuropsychiatr Dis Treat.* 2011;7:303-12.

200 Hoge EA, Worthington JJ, 3rd, Kaufman RE, Delong HR, Pollack MH, Simon NM. Aripiprazole as augmentation treatment of refractory generalized anxiety disorder and panic disorder. *CNS spectrums.* 2008;13(6):522-7.

201 Menza MA, Dobkin RD, Marin H. An open-label trial of aripiprazole augmentation for treatment-resistant generalized anxiety disorder. *Journal of clinical psychopharmacology.* 2007;27(2):207-10.

202 Stern RG, Petti TA, Bopp K, Tobia A. Aripiprazole for the treatment of schizophrenia with co-occurring social anxiety: an open-label cross-taper study. *Journal of clinical psychopharmacology.* 2009;29(3):206-9.

203 Shibasaki M, Kurokawa K, Mizuno K, Ohkuma S. Effect of aripiprazole on anxiety associated with ethanol physical dependence and on ethanol-induced place preference. *J Pharmacol Sci.* 2012;118(2):215-24.

204 Biojone C, Casarotto PC, Resstel LB, Zangrossi H, Jr., Guimaraes FS, Moreira FA. Anti-aversive effects of the atypical antipsychotic, aripiprazole, in animal models of anxiety. *Journal of psychopharmacology.* 2011;25(6):801-7.

205 Aripiprazole in the Treatment of Post-Traumatic Stress Disorder Symptoms. ClinicalTrials.gov [Internet]. Bethesda (MD): National Library of Medicine (US). 2007-[cited 2016 Jan 22]. https://clinicaltrials.gov/ct2/show/NCT00440713.

206 Aripiprazole in the Treatment of Patients With Schizophrenia and Symptoms of Obsessive Compulsive Disorder (OCD). ClinicalTrials.gov [Internet]. Bethesda (MD): National Library of Medicine (US). 2011-[cited 2016 Jan 22]. https://clinicaltrials.gov/ct2/show/NCT00374348.

207 Aripiprazole for the Treatment of Refractory Anxiety. ClinicalTrials.gov [Internet]. Bethesda (MD): National Library of Medicine (US). 2009-[cited 2016 Jan 22]. https://clinicaltrials.gov/ct2/show/NCT00438386.

208 Mailman RB, Murthy V. Third generation antipsychotic drugs: partial agonism or receptor functional selectivity? *Current pharmaceutical design.* 2010;16(5):488-501.

209 Strange PG. Antipsychotic drug action: antagonism, inverse agonism or partial agonism. *Trends Pharmacol Sci.* 2008;29(6):314-21.

210 Stahl SM. Dopamine system stabilizers, aripiprazole, and the next generation of antipsychotics, part 2: illustrating their mechanism of action. *The Journal of clinical psychiatry.* 2001;62(12):923-4.

211 Lieberman JA. Dopamine partial agonists: a new class of antipsychotic. *CNS drugs.* 2004;18(4):251-67.

212 Di Sciascio G, Riva MA. Aripiprazole: from pharmacological profile to clinical use. *Neuropsychiatr Dis Treat.* 2015;11:2635-47.

213 de Bartolomeis A, Tomasetti C, Iasevoli F. Update on the Mechanism of Action of Aripiprazole: Translational Insights into Antipsychotic Strategies Beyond Dopamine Receptor Antagonism. *CNS drugs.* 2015;29(9):773-99.

214 REXULTI- brexpiprazole tablet. DailyMed. Bethesda (MD): National Library of Medicine (US). http://dailymed.nlm.nih.gov/dailymed/drugInfo.cfm?id=5420.

215 Efficacy, Safety, and Tolerability of Brexpiprazole (OPC-34712) as Maintenance Treatment in Adults With Schizophrenia. ClinicalTrials.gov [Internet]. Bethesda (MD): National Library of Medicine (US). 2015-[cited 2016 Jan 22]. https://clinicaltrials.gov/ct2/show/NCT01668797.

216 Brexpiprazole in Patients With Schizophrenia. ClinicalTrials.gov [Internet]. Bethesda (MD): National Library of Medicine (US). 2016-[cited 2016 Jan 22]. https://clinicaltrials.gov/ct2/show/NCT01810783.

217 Study to Assess the Safety, Tolerability and Pharmacokinetics of Oral Brexpiprazole (OPC- 34712) in Adolescents With Schizophrenia. ClinicalTrials.gov [Internet]. Bethesda (MD): National Library of Medicine (US). 2016-[cited 2016 Jan 22]. https://clinicaltrials.gov/ct2/show/NCT02411695.

218 Citrome L, Stensbol TB, Maeda K. The preclinical profile of brexpiprazole: what is its clinical relevance for the treatment of psychiatric disorders? *Expert Rev Neurother.* 2015;15(10):1219-29.

219 McEvoy J, Citrome L. Brexpiprazole for the Treatment of Schizophrenia: A Review of this Novel Serotonin-Dopamine Activity Modulator. *Clin Schizophr Relat Psychoses.* 2016;9(4):177-86.

220 Correll CU, Skuban A, Ouyang J, Hobart M, Pfister S, McQuade RD, Nyilas M, Carson WH, Sanchez R, Eriksson H. Efficacy and Safety of Brexpiprazole for the Treatment of Acute Schizophrenia: A 6-Week Randomized, Double-Blind, Placebo-Controlled Trial. *The American journal of psychiatry.* 2015;172(9):870-80.

221 Kane JM, Skuban A, Ouyang J, Hobart M, Pfister S, McQuade RD, Nyilas M, Carson WH, Sanchez R, Eriksson H. A multicenter, randomized, double-blind, controlled phase 3 trial of fixed-dose brexpiprazole for the treatment of adults with acute schizophrenia. *Schizophrenia research.* 2015;164(1-3):127-35.

222 Thase ME, Youakim JM, Skuban A, Hobart M, Zhang P, McQuade RD, Nyilas M, Carson WH, Sanchez R, Eriksson H. Adjunctive brexpiprazole 1 and 3 mg for patients with major depressive disorder following inadequate response to antidepressants: a phase 3, randomized, double-blind study. *The Journal of clinical psychiatry.* 2015;76(9):1232-40.

223 Thase ME, Youakim JM, Skuban A, Hobart M, Augustine C, Zhang P, McQuade RD, Carson WH, Nyilas M, Sanchez R, Eriksson H. Efficacy and safety of adjunctive brexpiprazole 2 mg in major depressive disorder: a phase 3, randomized, placebo-controlled study in patients with inadequate response to antidepressants. *The Journal of clinical psychiatry.* 2015;76(9):1224-31.

224 Citrome L, Ota A, Nagamizu K, Perry P, et al. The effect of brexpiprazole (OPC-34712) versus aripiprazole in adult patients with acute schizophrenia: an exploratory study. 2015.

225 Dinama O, Warren AM, Kulkarni J. The role of pharmacogenomic testing in psychiatry: Real world examples. *Aust N Z J Psychiatry.* 2014;48(8):778.

226 Bertilsson L, Dahl ML, Dalen P, Al-Shurbaji A. Molecular genetics of CYP2D6: clinical relevance with focus on psychotropic drugs. *Br J Clin Pharmacol.* 2002;53(2):111-22.

227 Gaedigk A, Bradford LD, Marcucci KA, Leeder JS. Unique CYP2D6 activity distribution and genotype-phenotype discordance in black Americans. *Clin Pharmacol Ther.* 2002;72(1):76-89.

228 VRAYLAR- cariprazine capsule, gelatin coated DailyMed. Bethesda (MD): National Library of Medicine (US). http://dailymed.nlm.nih.gov/dailymed/drugInfo.cfm?id=5420.

229 Kane JM, Zukin S, Wang Y, Lu K, Ruth A, Nagy K, Laszlovszky I, Durgam S. Efficacy and Safety of Cariprazine in Acute Exacerbation of Schizophrenia: Results From an International, Phase III Clinical Trial. *Journal of clinical psychopharmacology.* 2015;35(4):367-73.

230 Calabrese JR, Keck PE, Jr., Starace A, Lu K, Ruth A, Laszlovszky I, Nemeth G, Durgam S. Efficacy and safety of low- and high-dose cariprazine in acute and mixed mania associated with bipolar I disorder: a double-blind, placebo-controlled study. *The Journal of clinical psychiatry.* 2015;76(3):284-92.

231 Sachs GS, Greenberg WM, Starace A, Lu K, Ruth A, Laszlovszky I, Nemeth G, Durgam S. Cariprazine in the treatment of acute mania in bipolar I disorder: a double-blind, placebo-controlled, phase III trial. *J Affect Disord.* 2015;174:296-302.

232 Durgam S, Starace A, Li D, Migliore R, Ruth A, Nemeth G, Laszlovszky I. The efficacy and tolerability of cariprazine in acute mania associated with bipolar I disorder: a phase II trial. *Bipolar Disord.* 2015;17(1):63-75.

233 Cariprazine Relative to Placebo in the Prevention of Relapse of Symptoms in Patients With Schizophrenia. ClinicalTrials.gov [Internet]. Bethesda (MD): National Library of Medicine (US). 2015-[cited 2016 Jan 22]. https://clinicaltrials.gov/ct2/show/NCT01412060.

234 Long-term Study of Cariprazine in Patients With Schizophrenia. ClinicalTrials.gov [Internet]. Bethesda (MD): National Library of Medicine (US). 2014-[cited 2016 Jan 22]. https://clinicaltrials.gov/ct2/show/NCT01104792.

235 The Purpose of the Study is to Determine Whether Cariprazine is a Safe and Tolerated Long-term Treatment in Patients With Chronic Stable Schizophrenia. ClinicalTrials.gov [Internet]. Bethesda (MD): National Library of Medicine (US). 2011-[cited 2016 Jan 22]. https://clinicaltrials.gov/ct2/show/NCT00839852.

236 Long-term Safety and Tolerability of Cariprazine for Bipolar I Disorder. ClinicalTrials.gov [Internet]. Bethesda (MD): National Library of Medicine (US). 2012-[cited 2016 Jan 22]. https://clinicaltrials.gov/ct2/show/NCT01059539.

237 Durgam S, Earley W, Lipschitz A, Guo H, Laszlovszky I, Nemeth G, Vieta E, Calabrese JR, Yatham LN. An 8-Week Randomized, Double-Blind, Placebo-Controlled Evaluation of the Safety and Efficacy of Cariprazine in Patients With Bipolar I Depression. *The American journal of psychiatry.* 2015;10.1176/appi.ajp.2015.15020164:appiajp201515020164.

238 Papp M, Gruca P, Lason-Tyburkiewicz M, Adham N, Kiss B, Gyertyan I. Attenuation of anhedonia by cariprazine in the chronic mild stress model of depression. *Behav Pharmacol.* 2014;25(5-6):567-74.

239 Safety, Tolerability, and Efficacy of Cariprazine in Patients With Bipolar Depression. ClinicalTrials.gov [Internet]. Bethesda (MD): National Library of Medicine (US). 2015-[cited 2016 Jan 22]. https://clinicaltrials.gov/ct2/show/NCT01396447.

240 Safety and Efficacy of RGH-188 (Cariprazine) in Bipolar Depression. ClinicalTrials.gov [Internet]. Bethesda (MD): National Library of Medicine (US). 2011-[cited 2016 Jan 22]. https://clinicaltrials.gov/ct2/show/NCT00852202.

241 Safety and Efficacy of Cariprazine as an Adjunctive to Antidepressant Therapy in Major Depressive Disorder. ClinicalTrials.gov [Internet]. Bethesda (MD): National Library of Medicine (US). 2014-[cited 2016 Jan 22]. https://clinicaltrials.gov/ct2/show/NCT01469377.

242 To Evaluate the Long-term Safety and Tolerability of Cariprazine as an Adjunctive Treatment to Antidepressant Therapy (ADT) in Patients With Major Depressive Disorder (MDD). ClinicalTrials.gov [Internet]. Bethesda (MD): National Library of Medicine (US). 2015-[cited 2016 Jan 22]. https://clinicaltrials.gov/ct2/show/NCT01838876.

243 Safety and Efficacy of Cariprazine As Adjunctive Therapy In Major Depressive Disorder. ClinicalTrials.gov [Internet]. Bethesda (MD): National Library of Medicine (US). 2012-[cited 2016 Jan 22]. https://clinicaltrials.gov/ct2/show/NCT00854100.

244 An Efficacy, Safety and Tolerability of Cariprazine as an Adjunctive Treatment to Antidepressant Therapy (ADT) in Patients With Major Depressive Disorder (MDD). ClinicalTrials.gov [Internet]. Bethesda (MD): National Library of Medicine (US). 2015-[cited 2016 Jan 22]. https://clinicaltrials.gov/ct2/show/NCT01715805.

245 Caccia S, Invernizzi RW, Nobili A, Pasina L. A new generation of antipsychotics: pharmacology and clinical utility of cariprazine in schizophrenia. *Ther Clin Risk Manag.* 2013;9:319-28.

246 Stahl SM. Multifunctional drugs: a novel concept for psychopharmacology. *CNS spectrums.* 2009;14(2):71-3.

247 DeVane CL, Nemeroff CB. Clinical pharmacokinetics of quetiapine: an atypical antipsychotic. *Clin Pharmacokinet.* 2001;40(7):509-22.

248 Grunder G. Cariprazine, an orally active D2/D3 receptor antagonist, for the potential treatment of schizophrenia, bipolar mania and depression. *Curr Opin Investig Drugs.* 2010;11(7):823-32.

249 Citrome L. Cariprazine: chemistry, pharmacodynamics, pharmacokinetics, and metabolism, clinical efficacy, safety, and tolerability. *Expert Opin Drug Metab Toxicol.* 2013;9(2):193-206.

250 Gyertyan I, Kiss B, Saghy K, Laszy J, Szabo G, Szabados T, Gemesi LI, Pasztor G, Zajer-Balazs M, Kapas M, Csongor EA, Domany G, Tihanyi K, Szombathelyi Z. Cariprazine (RGH-188), a potent D3/D2 dopamine receptor partial agonist, binds to dopamine D3 receptors in vivo and shows antipsychotic-like and procognitive effects in rodents. *Neurochem Int.* 2011;59(6):925-35.

TABLES

Table 1. Treatment indications and recommended dosing strategies of the '-done' second generation antipsychotics. The FDA approved treatment indications and dosing strategies (initial dose, titration and dose adjustment, target dose, and maximum recommended dose) for each unique agent are listed. *Denotes a black box warning of increased mortality in elderly patients with dementia-related psychosis. †Denotes a black box warning of increased suicidality with concomitant use of antidepressants in children and young adults. Unless otherwise specified, all dosing strategy data was garnered from regulatory package inserts[50,84,88,112,122,140,161,176,187,214,228]. Abbreviations: bid, twice daily.

Table 1

	Approved Treatment Indications		Initial Dose	Titration	Target Dose	Maximum Dose
Risperidone*	Schizophrenia: acute and maintenance	Adults	2.0 mg/day	1.0-2.0 mg/day	4.0-8.0 mg/day	16.0 mg/day
		Adolescents (13-17 years)	0.5 mg/day	0.5-1.0 mg/day	3.0 mg/day	6.0 mg/day
	Bipolar I Disorder: acute manic or mixed episode	Adults (monotherapy or adjunct)	2.0-3.0 mg/day	1.0 mg/day	3.0 mg/day	6.0 mg/day
		Adolescents (10-17 years; adjunct)	0.5 mg/day	0.5-1.0 mg/day	2.5 mg/day	6.0 mg/day
	Autism: irritability and aggression	Adolescents (5-16 years)	0.25-0.5 mg/day	0.5-1.0 mg/14 days	0.5-2.5 mg/day	3.0 mg/day
Paliperidone*	Schizophrenia: acute and maintenance	Adults	6.0 mg/day	3.0 mg/5 days	6.0 mg/day	12.0 mg/day
		Adolescents (12-17 years)	3.0 mg/day	3.0 mg/5 days	3.0 mg/day	6.0 mg/day
	Schizoaffective disorder	Adults (monotherapy or adjunct)	6.0 mg/day	3.0 mg/4 days	6.0 mg/day	12.0 mg/day
Ziprasidone*	Schizophrenia: acute and maintenance	Adults	20.0 mg bid	20.0 mg bid/2 days	20.0-80.0 mg bid	100.0 mg bid
	Schizophrenia: acute agitation	Adults (IM injection)	10.0-20.0 mg	10.0 mg every 2 hr or 20.0 mg every 4 hr	-	40.0 mg/day
	Bipolar I Disorder: acute manic or mixed episode	Adults (monotherapy)	40.0 mg bid	60.0-80.0 mg bid on second day	40.0-80.0 mg bid	100.0 mg bid
	Bipolar I Disorder: maintenance	Adults (adjunct)	Same as acute	Same as acute	Same as acute	Same as acute
Iloperidone*	Schizophrenia: acute	Adults	1.0 mg bid	2.0, 4.0, 6.0, 8.0, 10.0, 12.0 mg bid on days 2, 3, 4, 5, 6, and 7	6.0-12.0 mg bid	12 mg bid
Lurasidone*†	Schizophrenia: acute	Adults	40.0 mg/day	-	40.0-160.0 mg/day	160.0 mg/day
	Bipolar I Disorder: depressive episodes	Adults (monotherapy or adjunct)	20.0 mg/day	-	20.0-60.0.0 mg/day	120.0 mg/day

Table 2. Treatment indications and recommended dosing strategies of the '-pine' second generation antipsychotics. The FDA approved treatment indications and dosing strategies (initial dose, titration and dose adjustment, target dose, and maximum recommended dose) for each unique agent are listed. *Denotes a black box warning of increased mortality in elderly patients with dementia-related psychosis. †Denotes a black box warning of increased suicidality with concomitant use of antidepressants in children and young adults. Unless otherwise specified, all dosing strategy data was garnered from regulatory package inserts[50,84,88,112,122,140,161,176,187,214,228]. Abbreviations: bid, twice daily.

Table 2

	Approved Treatment Indications		Initial Dose	Titration	Target Dose	Maximum Dose
Olanzapine*†	Schizophrenia: acute and maintenance	Adults	5.0-10.0 mg/day	5.0 mg/1 week	10.0 mg/day	20.0 mg/day
		Adolescent (13-17 years)	2.5-5.0 mg/day	2.5-5.0 mg/1 week	10.0 mg/day	20.0 mg/day
	Bipolar I Disorder: acute mania or mixed episode	Adults (monotherapy or adjunct)	10.0-15.0 mg/day	5.0 mg/day	10.0-15.0 mg/day	20.0 mg/day
		Adolescent (13-17 years; monotherapy)	2.5-5.0 mg/day	2.5-5.0 mg/day	10.0 mg/day	20.0 mg/day
	Bipolar I Disorder: maintenance	Adults (monotherapy)	Same as acute	Same as acute	Same as acute	Same as acute
	Schizophrenia or Bipolar Mania: acute agitation	Adults (IM injection)	2.5-10.0 mg	2.5-10.0 mg 2-4 hr apart	10.0 mg	30.0 mg/day
	Bipolar I Disorder: acute depressive episode	Adults (olanzapine/fluoxetine)	6.0/25.0 mg/day	3.0/25.0 mg/1 week	6.0-12.0/25.0-50.0 mg/day	18.0/75.0 mg/day
	Bipolar I Disorder: acute depressive episode	Adolescent (10-17 years)	3.0/25.0 mg/day	3.0/25.0 mg/1 week	6.0-12.0/25.0-50.0 mg/day	12.0/50.0 mg/day
	Major Depressive Disorder: treatment resistant	Adults (olanzapine/fluoxetine)	6.0/25.0 mg/day	3.0/25.0 mg/1 week	6.0-18.0/25.0-50.0 mg/day	18.0/75.0 mg/day
Quetiapine*†	Schizophrenia: acute and maintenance	Adults	300.0 mg/day	50.0-300.0 mg/day	400.0-800.0 mg/day	800.0 mg/day
		Adolescent (13-17 years)	50.0 mg/day	100.0, 200.0, 300.0, 400.0 mg/day on days 2, 3, 4, and 5	400.0-800.0 mg/day	800.0 mg/day
	Bipolar I Disorder: acute mania or mixed episode	Adults (monotherapy or adjunct)	300.0 mg/day	600.0 mg/day on day 2, 400.0-800.0 mg/day on day 3	400.0-800.0 mg/day	800.0 mg/day
		Adolescent (10-17 years; monotherapy)	50.0 mg/day	100.0, 200.0, 300.0, 400.0 mg/day on days 2, 3, 4, and 5	400.0-600.0 mg/day	600.0 mg/day
	Bipolar I Disorder: maintenance	Adults (adjunct)	Same as acute	Same as acute	Same as acute	Same as acute
	Bipolar I Disorder: acute depressive episode	Adults (monotherapy)	50.0 mg/day	100.0, 200.0, 300.0 mg/day on days 2, 3, and 4	300.0 mg/day	300.0 mg/day
	Major Depressive Disorder	Adults (adjunct)	50.0 mg/day	50.0 mg/day on day 2, 150.0 mg/day on day 3	150.0-300.0 mg/day	300.0 mg/day
Asenapine*	Schizophrenia: acute	Adults	5.0 mg bid	5.0 mg bid/1 week	5.0 mg bid	10.0 mg bid
	Bipolar I Disorder: acute mania or mixed episode	Adults (monotherapy or adjunct)	10.0 mg bid	-	5.0-10.0 mg bid	10.0 mg bid
		Adolescents (10-17 years; monotherapy)	2.5 mg bid	5.0 mg bid (day 3); 10.0 mg bid (day 6)	2.5-10.0 mg bid	10.0 mg bid

Table 3. Treatment indications and recommended dosing strategies of the '-pip' and '-rip' second generation antipsychotics. The FDA approved treatment indications and dosing strategies (initial dose, titration and dose adjustment, target dose, and maximum recommended dose) for each unique agent are listed. *Denotes a black box warning of increased mortality in elderly patients with dementia-related psychosis. †Denotes a black box warning of increased suicidality with concomitant use of antidepressants in children and young adults. Unless otherwise specified, all dosing strategy data was garnered from regulatory package inserts[50,84,88,112,122,140,161,176,187,214,228]. Abbreviations: bid, twice daily.

Table 3

	Approved Treatment Indications		Initial Dose	Titration	Target Dose	Maximum Dose
Aripiprazole*†	Schizophrenia: acute and maintenance	Adults	10.0-15.0 mg/day	5.0 mg/2 weeks	10.0-15.0 mg/day	30.0 mg/day
		Adolescents (13-17 years)	2.0 mg/day	5.0 mg/day on day 2, 10.0 mg/day on day 4, 5.0 mg/2 weeks thereafter	10.0 mg/day	30.0 mg/day
	Bipolar I Disorder: acute manic or mixed episode	Adults (monotherapy or adjunct)	10.0-15.0 mg/day	5.0 mg/2 weeks	15.0 mg/day	30.0 mg/day
		Adolescents (10-17 years; monotherapy or adunct)	2.0 mg/day	5.0 mg/day on day 2, 10.0 mg/day on day 4, 5.0 mg/2 weeks thereafter	10.0 mg/day	30.0 mg/day
	Bipolar I Disorder: maintenance	Adults (monotherapy or adjunct)	Same as acute	Same as acute	Same as acute	Same as acute
		Adolescents (10-17 years; monotherapy or adunct)	Same as acute	Same as acute	Same as acute	Same as acute
	Schizophrenia or Bipolar Mania: acute agitation	Adults (IM injection)	9.75 mg	Every 2 hours as needed	5.25-15.0 mg	30.0 mg/day
	Major Depressive Disorder	Adults (adjunct)	2.0-5.0 mg/day	5.0 mg/1 week	2.0-15.0 mg/day	15.0 mg/day
	Autism: irritability and aggression	Adolescents (6-17 years)	2.0 mg/day	5.0 mg/1 week	5.0-15.0 mg/day	15.0 mg/day
	Tourette's Disorder	Adolescents (6-18 years)	2.0 mg/day	5.0 mg/day on day 2, 5.0 mg/1 week thereafter	5.0-20.0 mg/day	20.0 mg/day
Brexpiprazole*†	Schizophrenia: acute	Adults	1.0 mg/day	2.0 mg/day on day 5, 4.0 mg on day 8	2.0-4.0 mg/day	4.0 mg/day
	Major Depressive Disorder	Adults (adjunct)	0.5-1.0 mg/day	0.5-1.0 mg/1 week	2.0 mg/day	3.0 mg/day
Cariprazine*†	Schizophrenia: acute	Adults	1.5 mg/day	3.0 mg/day on day 2, 1.5-3.0 mg/several weeks	1.5-6.0 mg/day	6.0 mg/day
	Bipolar I Disorder: acute mania or mixed episode	Adults (monotherapy)	1.5 mg/day	3.0 mg/day on day 2, 1.5-3.0 mg/several weeks	3.0-6.0 mg/day	6.0 mg/day

Table 4. Pharmacokinetics of the second generation antipsychotics. Parameters represented included oral bioavailability, time to peak plasma concentration, half-life, time to steady-state concentration, and the major cytochrome P450 (CYP) isoenzymes responsible for metabolism. *Denotes that based upon oral bioavailability, the only two antipsychotics currently recommended to take with food are ziprasidone and lurasidone (at least 350 kcal). †Denotes that sublingual asenapine tablets require no food or drink up to 15 minutes after administration to ensure proper absorption. [A]In a food effect study, C_{max} and area under the curve (AUC) were 3- and 2-times higher, respectively, when given with food versus fasting conditions[125]. [B]Although not listed in the online packet insert[140], according to 'Applied Pharmacokinetics & Pharmacodynamics: Principles of Therapeutic Drug Monitoring', the bioavailability of olanzapine is 87.0%[141]. [C]Although one source claims the absolute oral bioavailability of quetiapine is unknown, it states the relative bioavailability from orally administered tablets compared to solution was almost complete[247]. However, another study using lipid nanoparticles to improve the oral bioavailability of quetiapine claimed that due to extensive first-pass metabolism, there is a poor bioavailability of 9% associated with this drug[162]. There was no mention of the oral bioavailability in the regulatory package insert[161]. [D]An oral bioavailability of cariprazine could not be found in the online packet insert or relevant pharmacokinetic literature, only stated as being 'high'[228,248,249]. A study in rats demonstrated an oral bioavailabilty of 52% at a dose of 1.0 mg/kg[250]. Unless otherwise specified, all pharmacokinetic data was garnered from regulatory package inserts[50,84,88,112,122,140,161,176,187,214,228].

Table 4

	Oral Bioavailability (%)	Oral Bioavailability: With Food (%)	Time to Peak Plasma Concentration (hours)	Half Life (hours)	Time to Steady State Concentration (days)	CYP450 Metabolism
Risperidone	70.0	-	1.0-2.0	3.0	1.0	CYP2D6
Paliperidone	28.0	42.0	24.0	24.0	4.0-5.0	-
Ziprasidone*	-	60.0	6.0-8.0	7.0	1.0-3.0	CYP3A4
Iloperidone	96.0	-	2.0-4.0	18.0	3.0-4.0	CYP2D6, CYP3A4
Lurasidone*	9.0-19.0	18.0-38.0[A]	1.0-3.0	18.0	7.0	CYP3A4
Olanzapine	87.0[B]	-	6.0	30.0	7.0	CYP2D6, CYP1A2
Quetiapine	9.0[C]	-	6.0	7.0	2.0	CYP3A4
Asenapine†	35.0	-	0.5-1.5	24.0	3.0	CYP1A2
Aripiprazole	87.0	-	3.0-5.0	75.0	14.0	CYP2D6, CYP3A4
Brexpiprazole	95.0	-	4.0	91.0	10.0-12.0	CYP2D6, CYP3A4
Cariprazine	High[D]	-	3.0-6.0	48.0-96.0	7.0-14.0	CYP3A4

Table 5. Binding affinity profiles of the second generation antipsychotics. The unique pharmacodynamic profiles (as measured by binding affinity, or Ki) for each of the current second generation antipsychotics at each receptor site are listed in a columnar format. Unless otherwise specified, columns represent antagonism at these specific receptor sites. *Denotes partial agonism at that receptor site, while † represents inhibition. Norquetiapine, the main active metabolite of quietiapine is also included, due to its striking difference in pharmacodynamic profile from the parent drug. 'X': little-to-no binding affinity (Ki > 1,000). '+': weak binding affinity (100 > Ki < 1,000). '++': moderate binding affinity (10 > Ki < 100). '+++': strong binding affinity (1.0 > Ki < 10). '++++': very strong binding affinity (0.1 > Ki < 1.0). '+++++': extremely strong binding affinity (Ki < 0.1). All Ki values were garnered from regulatory package inserts[50,84,88,112,122,140,161,176,187,214,228]. Abbreviations: D2, dopamine D2 receptor; D3, dopamine D3 receptor; 5-HT1a, serotonin 1a receptor; 5-HT2a, serotonin 2a receptor; 5-HT2c, serotonin 2c receptor; 5-HT6, serotonin 6 receptor; 5-HT7, serotonin 7 receptor; α1, alpha adrenergic 1 receptor; α2, alpha adrenergic 2 receptor; M1, muscarinic acetylcholine 1 receptor; H1, histamine 1 receptor; NET, norepinephrine transporter; SERT, serotonin transporter.

Table 5

	D2	D2*	D3	D3*	5-HT1a*	5-HT2a	5-HT2c	5-HT6	5-HT7	α1	α2	M1	H1	NET†	SERT†
Risperidone	+++		++		+	++++	++	X	+++	+++	+++	X	++	X	X
Paliperidone	+++		+++		X	++++	++	X	+++	+++	+++	X	++	X	X
Ziprasidone	+++		+++		+++	++++	+++	++	+++	+++	+	X	++	++	+
Iloperidone	++		+++		+	+++	+	++	+++	++++	+	X	+	X	
Lurasidone	++++				+++	++++	+		++++	++	++	X	X		
Olanzapine	++		++		X	+++	++	++	+	++	+	++	+++	X	X
Quetiapine	+		+		X	++	X	X	+	++	X	X	+++	X	X
Norquetiapine	+		+		+	+++	++++	+	+++	+++	X	++	+++	++	+
Asenapine	+++		++++		+++	+++++	+++++	++++	+++	+++	+++	X	+++		
Aripiprazole		++++		+++	+++	+++	++	+	++	++	++	X	++	X	++
Brexpiprazole		++++		+++	++++	++++	++		+++	+++		X	++		
Cariprazine		++++		+++++	+++	++	+	X	+	+	X	X	++		X

89